# Praise for
## ROAD MAP TO HOLLAND

❧

"Rich with honesty, wisdom, and a deep appreciation for every-day miracles, *Road Map to Holland* is a thoughtful, moving med-itation on the struggles and joys Jennifer Graf Groneberg and her family experienced during her son Avery's first two years. Groneberg offers a wealth of insight, information, and even prac-tical resources for families whose children have Down syndrome. Yet this book is first and foremost a story about the constant discovery of love, and it will resonate with every reader who has traveled the always unpredictable, often overwhelming, wonder-filled journey into parenthood."

—Kim Edwards, author of *The Memory Keeper's Daughter*

"What a remarkable book! With excruciating candor and exqui-site generosity, Jennifer Graf Groneberg invites us into the deep-est privacy of her innermost thoughts, feelings, fears, challenges, and triumphs. Nothing is left out in this amazingly intimate and profound journal. She allows us into every nook and cranny of her life, and we find ourselves firmly ensconced in her heart."

—Emily Perl Kingsley, national spokesperson and advocate for people with disabilities and author of "Welcome to Holland"

"This is the story of Avery—a child with Down syndrome who transformed his mother's broken heart into one filled with cheer, awe, and pride. He offers all new and expectant parents a powerful perspective on life's greatest lessons."

—Brian Skotko, M.D., M.P.P., Children's Hospital Boston and Boston Medical Center

*continued . . .*

# ROAD MAP TO HOLLAND

How I Found My Way Through
My Son's First Two Years
with Down Syndrome

Jennifer Graf Groneberg

 NEW AMERICAN LIBRARY

New American Library
Published by New American Library,
a division of Penguin Group (USA) Inc.,
375 Hudson Street, New York, New York 10014, USA
Penguin Group (Canada), 90 Eglinton Avenue East, Suite 700, Toronto,
Ontario M4P 2Y3, Canada (a division of Pearson Penguin Canada Inc.)
Penguin Books Ltd., 80 Strand, London WC2R 0RL, England
Penguin Ireland, 25 St. Stephen's Green, Dublin 2,
Ireland (a division of Penguin Books Ltd.)
Penguin Group (Australia), 250 Camberwell Road, Camberwell,
Victoria 3124, Australia (a division of Pearson Australia Group Pty. Ltd.)
Penguin Books India Pvt. Ltd., 11 Community Centre,
Panchsheel Park, New Delhi – 110 017, India
Penguin Group (NZ), 67 Apollo Drive, Rosedale, North Shore 0632,
New Zealand (a division of Pearson New Zealand Ltd.)
Penguin Books (South Africa) (Pty.) Ltd., 24 Sturdee Avenue,
Rosebank, Johannesburg 2196, South Africa

Penguin Books Ltd., Registered Offices:
80 Strand, London WC2R 0RL, England

First published by New American Library,
a division of Penguin Group (USA) Inc.

First Printing, April 2008
10  9  8  7  6  5  4  3

"Late Fragment" from *A New Path to the Waterfall* by Raymond Carver. Copyright © 1989 by
the Estate of Raymond Carver. Used by permission of Gove/Atlantic, Inc.
"Welcome to Holland" by Emily Perl Kingsley. Copyright © Emily Perl Kingsley, 1987. All
rights reserved. Reprinted by permission of the author.

REGISTERED TRADEMARK—MARCA REGISTRADA

LIBRARY OF CONGRESS CATALOGING-IN-PUBLICATION DATA:
Groneberg, Jennifer Graf.
Road map to Holland: how i found my way through my son's first two years with Down
syndrome/Jennifer Graf Groneberg.
p.  cm.
ISBN: 978-0-451-22295-4
1. Groneberg, Jennifer Graf. 2. Groneberg, Bennett. 3. Mothers of children with disabilities—
United States—Biography. 4. Down syndrome—Patients—United States—Biography. 5. Down
syndrome—Patients—United States—Family relationships. I. Title.
RJ506.D68G74 2008
618.92'858842092—dc22        2007033444 [B]

Set in Stempel Garamond  •  Designed by Elke Sigal

Printed in the United States of America

*For our children*

# Acknowledgments

There's an adage that it takes a village to raise a child—I'm tempted to say the same is true for writing a book, but in my case, it's more like a small metropolis. My helpers came from far and wide, and in naming them all, I realize my only claim to this book is that I brought the words. Many others contributed essentials, including:

My mom, Christine Graf, who saved everything I ever wrote, some of it in picture frames. My dad and his wife, Fred and Pam Graf, who encouraged me to dream big dreams. Don and Joyce Groneberg: I'd have married Tom just to become part of his family. Bob and Elizabeth Groneberg, and Denys and Glynnis Slater, aunts and uncles to my children. My grandparents, June and John Vincent, and my writing fairy godmothers, Laurie Buehler and Sara Esgate.

Laura Nolan, for the pleasure of a thirty-year friendship and for finding exactly the right home for my words, and my editor, Tracy Bernstein, who is gentle, kind, wise, and firm. She's the kind of mother you'd want for your children, and she shared her talents as a second mother to this book.

Whenever I lost my way, Claudia Cunningham reassured me by saying, "Tell them what you saw. That's all you have to do." Phyllis Walker wrapped my first draft in a pink-and-blue ribbon;

she's the midwife of this story. And Sarah Smith, who introduces me as "my friend, the author." Thank you for believing it.

Emily River, bearer of many gifts, including, at the finish line, a lobster dinner flown in from the East Coast. Nicole Tavenner took beautiful photographs of my family. Judith Bromley told me, "You have to write this book. I will help you," then proceeded to feed me encouragement, pasta in red sauce, and coffee brownies, as needed.

And the Wildhorse Writer's Group—Judith, Claudia, Phyllis, and Gary Acevedo, Cindy Doll, Mary Gertson, JoAnne Hines, Jackie Ladner, Milana Marsenich, Angela Nolan, Maggie Plummer, Julie Wenner—you brought kindness and suggested revisions in perfect measure.

Others, too: Vicki Forman, Kathy Soper, Sue Robins, Rebecca Phong, Jennifer Enderlin. Mary Cross and Mary Ann McGowan. Wendy Sitter, Molly Beck, Brittney Bennetts. You've blessed me with your friendship and support.

Kristin Darguzas at ParentDish gave me a place to tell my Avery stories; Amy Anderson and Sheri Reed welcomed me to mamazine.com with open arms. BabyCenter.com, Downsyn.com, T21 Online, and Uno Mas!—all groups of extraordinary people who've created places where everyone is welcome and no one ever has to explain.

And finally, Tom, who believed I could do it, and Carter, Avery, and Bennett, who show me how every day.

# Contents

*Sunday's child is full of grace.*

# 1

## At First, It Hurts to Breathe

It's hard to know where to begin.

It might start five days after the end of my second pregnancy. I am in the Neonatal Intensive Care Unit (NICU) with my mother-in-law, Joyce, and we have just finished holding the babies. In the ten seconds that follow, my life changes so completely and thoroughly that for a while I am unable to speak.

Our pediatrician is Dr. Rosquist, a woman my age who, under other circumstances, might have been a friend. Lean and light, fair-skinned, with almost white hair, she reminds me of lemon sherbet. When I've returned Avery to his isolette, tucked Bennett back into his green-and-yellow knit cap, and handed him to his nurse to be weighed, she comes over to us. She sits down next to me, reaches out, and touches my forearm. I know that whatever she has to tell me is going to be bad.

But I should begin earlier. It would have been a busy morning in the NICU, as that is when Dr. Rosquist, first name Jennifer, like mine, makes her rounds. The room would have been noisy, filled with the hum of the HVAC, the clicking of the fluorescent lights overhead, the near-constant beeping of the pulse-oxygen monitors, an occasional alarm, but in my mind it is still—all the sound quieting to the small, irregular breathing of my son Avery as she examines him. Stethoscope to the palm of her hand to warm it, hands inside the isolette touching him, stethoscope on his heart. Is it the shape of his head that catches her eye, or ears placed slightly too low, or a particular crease in the palm of his left hand? On the clipboard at the base of his isolette, she writes a note to herself, a reminder to order a blood draw to be sent away to Shodair Children's Hospital for a test.

Earlier still, there's the moment the babies are pulled out of me seven weeks premature. An emergency C-section performed by a doctor I don't know, in a hospital seventy-five miles from home. Eyes peering over blue surgical masks, the members of my "team," who assembled at a moment's notice on a bright, sunny Sunday in June. The nurse who talks me through the procedure is gentle; the soft blue of her scrubs reminds me of the Pacific Ocean, which I knew as a girl. The babies come quickly; pulled out by a man I call Doc Hollywood after his long thick hair, his tan, his Hawaiian scrubs, which are novelties where I live, a small mountain town in northwest Montana. He is confident and extraordinarily kind. He holds up the first baby, Baby A, our Avery, and says, "What a beautiful boy. Congratulations." Then comes his twin, Baby B, Bennett. "Another healthy boy. Way to go, Mom." The cries of newborns fill the room, the hearty sounds of my new sons.

But there is a beginning even before that, a snowy evening in late October when my husband, Tom, and I pile extra wood in the stove to bank it against the night, tuck three-year-old Carter into bed, and find ourselves with a quiet house and a moment alone together. We'd been trying to have a second child for almost a year, timing our lives to the rhythms of my cycle, and the months had taken their toll. Sadly, we had begun letting go of the idea that there would be more babies for us—we join together that blustery night simply out of love for each other. Sometime in the predawn, two lives take root inside me, not one baby but two, a prayer that we hadn't even spoken, answered. Cells multiplying and dividing, a frenzy of growth and activity, whole lives changing forever, all while I sleep curled into my pillow, my back against Tom's, both of us warm in the thick down comforter, as the snow continues to blow well past sunrise.

These are the instances that define Avery's birth, but I could go back in time further. There is the first wailing breath I took as a pink-haired baby, born five weeks early to a young husband and wife who were slightly bewildered by my arrival but game to give it a go as a family nevertheless. Or the night they met as freshmen on a small Midwestern college campus. My mom, my dad, barely out of high school and each on their own for the first time. Mom was a cheerleader, Dad was a football player, and though they had noticed each other around campus, they met officially at a fall mixer. A simple glance, an innocent smile, the beginning of a flirtation that would lead to a life together and two children, both daughters, who would later become the mothers of sons.

All the children a woman will bear are present inside her even before she is born. They are created while she is still nothing more than a tiny form twisting and floating in utero. For a time, three generations—mother, daughter, and granddaughter—live as one. It is a matriarchal line. My mother was the second daughter in a matriarchal line noted for twin births. My grandmother, with each of her three pregnancies, had wished for twins. She never got them, and her children never delivered twins, so she thought the tendency had ended with her.

My father is the second son in his family. The first baby, his older brother, was sickly, and had medical complications through-out his life. He died of natural causes when he was in his twenties, a short lifetime but one that exceeded all expectations. His name was David. This is all I know. What happened to him, and why, is not often talked about in my father's family. What is discussed is that I resemble my father's mother, my grandmother. We share many traits: light brown curly hair; pale blue eyes; a similar button nose; a tendency to grow round and full—sturdy, farmwife stock.

Two grandmothers, a mother and father, me; a blustery fall day, a twin pregnancy, a premature delivery. The babies in the hospital, seemingly fine, but no, perhaps there is something more. A request for a blood draw. All of these events connect. Each is a link, one to another, in the long, twisted chain of my son's DNA. If you stretch it end to end, it would reach to the moon. A son I had wished for, yearned for, and yet when he arrives, I'm wholly unprepared, despite all the reasons I should have known better.

Dr. Rosquist is in the NICU in the afternoon, which is not her usual time. I'm holding Avery. Joyce is holding Bennett. When we return them to their isolettes, the doctor comes over to us. She pulls up a chair next to my rocker, reaches out, touches my arm. "I have some news," she says, glancing over at Joyce.

"It's okay. Joyce can stay," I say.

"It's the results of the FISH test," she says.

I clearly remember her ordering it. She'd had some concerns. Little things, like the way Avery's ears looked and a tiny crease in his left palm.

She unfolds a piece of paper. In front of me is a photocopy of pairs of squiggly lines that represent chromosomes. Of each pair, one comes from the father, one from the mother. It is a map of sorts, a map of genetic destiny.

My eyes scan the paper—dots and squiggles, two by two, until there, I see something different. An extra dot. At the twenty-first pair of chromosomes, Avery has one extra. Where there should be two, there are three.

"What does this mean?" I mumble.

"Avery has Down syndrome."

"But what does this mean?" I repeat, this time a little louder. Words, which usually come so easily, are failing me. I want to know what's going to happen to us. What will happen to Avery? To Bennett, to Carter? I want reassurance that we will all be okay.

"What does it mean?" I ask again, feeling as if I were suddenly speaking the wrong language. The doctor's demeanor, the sadness in her eyes, tells me it is something bad. *Broken,* I think. *She's telling me my baby is broken.*

There is an awful silence, in which the world I know spins away from me and I'm left alone, stunned and speechless. There is the hum of the HVAC, the clicking of the fluorescent lights overhead, the near-constant beeping of the pulse-oxygen monitors, the occasional alarm. I can't find enough air, can't draw it in deeply enough. No matter how many times I inhale, I can't catch my breath.

I have an overpowering desire to flee. To get up and run, away from the stale air, the unnatural light, the metallic smell of blood and bleach and my own fear. I could start over, be someone else, anyone but who I am, anyone but the mother of two babies trapped in plastic boxes in the NICU. And now one of them is not right, lost, gone.

I could find a motel room and sleep for days. I'd get on the highway and drive east, toward the night, toward the city, a woman with a secret past, abandoned children, an ex-life. Even as I feel a shiver run through my legs, I know I'll never do it. My babies, my love, a life I could never leave.

I nod my head mutely, dumbly, up and down, up and down. It means "Yes," it means "I understand," it means "I can't think of anything else to do." My eyes well with tears, and I don't know whom I am crying for, Avery or myself. It all seems like too much to bear. Joyce pats my knee. Dr. Rosquist asks if I have any other questions. I still can't speak. I have no idea what to do. And then it comes to me. I want to hold Avery.

I point to his isolette, my hand shaking.

"Get Avery?" Dr. Rosquist asks.

I nod yes.

A nurse appears out of nowhere, but Dr. Rosquist waves her aside. She unlatches the top of the box and carefully lifts Avery up and into my arms. He is pink and red and blotchy, like most newborns. He has a little tuft of downy brown hair. I can't see anything wrong with him. For a fleeting moment, I think perhaps it's all a mistake. But no, there are the papers and their unmistakable black-and-white truth. I look into Avery's eyes. They are deep, dark blue like a lake on a stormy day. Around the irises are tiny white spots that glitter. They are the most beautiful eyes I've ever seen.

"Hello," I manage to whisper through my tears, as if meeting him for the first time. "Hello." I pull him close and rock too fast, too hard, and he begins to cry, too. Both of us crying and rocking, his little hand wrapped tight around my thumb.

We stay like this for a while, or a thousand whiles—I lose track of time. Soon enough he is asleep in my arms, and it is time for Joyce and me to go. I slide my thumb out from his fist, gently place him back in his isolette, and whisper good-bye to both babies. Joyce follows me. At the exit, we pull off our hospital gowns and toss them in the laundry bin. While we are leaving, a nurse I have never seen comes up to me.

"I wanted to tell you," she says, "there's a waiting list for babies like yours. People wait in line to adopt them."

I don't understand her meaning. Is that what people do? Do they give their babies to families who know about Down syndrome? Is that the thing to do? I'm too tired to think about it. All I want to do is sleep, perhaps for the rest of my life.

Outside the NICU, Joyce gives me a hug.

"Are you hungry?" she asks.

"I guess I probably should eat," I say. I'm pumping breast milk for the babies every three hours, and I want to keep my milk up. But I don't feel hungry.

We walk to the hospital cafeteria. I select a turkey sandwich.

Joyce has tuna. We eat in silence. I don't know what she is thinking or feeling, because I am so lost in my own sadness. And Joyce is the kind of person who knows when to talk about something and when not to talk about something. She is giving me space to figure out what I'm feeling.

I'm thinking about how quickly everything can change—only a few hours earlier, I'd been worried about Bennett, because he was the one who was having trouble keeping his milk down. Tom and I had thought of Avery as the tough, strong baby, and Bennett as the weaker one. We'd joked Avery would be a football player, he was growing so fast.

Two words changed all that.

I wonder what else is going on in this hospital cafeteria—who else has heard words that changed their lives completely? I take comfort in the thought that I'm probably not the only one in the room gripped by a sadness so powerful it feels physical, as if I've been stripped of my skin, left raw and open. It hurts to chew, to swallow. It even hurts to breathe.

We finish our sandwiches and find our way to the car. Joyce is driving, since I am still recovering from the C-section. I ask her if she feels steady enough.

"Oh, yes, I'll be fine," she says.

I open the passenger-side door and here it comes, another wave of grief. This is the car we'd bought after the ultrasound had shown two babies. It's a white '97 Ford Expedition, one of the few models that holds three car seats in the back.

I remember the day we bought it, me so big and round, waddling from car to car, peering into each backseat, saying, "No, too small." I was stalling. I didn't see why we needed a new car. Our old one was fine. But Tom was insistent—we needed a safe place to put three car seats.

All our hopes, all our dreams, broken. This wasn't how it was supposed to be: babies born too early, the NICU, and now Avery.

I'd had a normal pregnancy, in the beginning. I felt a seasick kind of nausea that was worse than the morning sickness with my first baby, but I'd heard no two pregnancies were alike. I seemed to grow faster, too, but I'd been told that was to be expected with second pregnancies. My doctor was a great Clydesdale of a woman with a big smile and an easy laugh. During a routine appointment, she looked up and, with a little catch in her throat, said quickly, "We should schedule an ultrasound as soon as we can." I stared back at her across the white expanse of my belly, the worry already starting. She laughed her big laugh and explained, "I want to get a look. Are you sure about your dates?" I was. The other possibilities ranged from multiple fetuses to complications I didn't want to imagine—tumors, excess amniotic fluid, or worse. The next day, with Tom by my side, the ultrasound technician, a thin woman named Tally, looked up from the hazy black-and-white image on the monitor and said, "Two."

Even the thought of it, of those times that now seem so innocent, sends me back to crying. I manage to pull myself into the seat and buckle the belt. Joyce pauses, reaches over to me, takes my hand, and squeezes it. It feels unusual to be holding hands with my mother-in-law, but it feels safe. She looks at me and says, "You take it one day at a time. That's what you do. One day at a time." She lets go of my hand, then turns the key, and the engine comes to life. She puts the car into gear and pulls out of the parking lot. She drives, and I feel like a little girl sitting in the passenger seat.

Her gentleness, her steadfastness, and her faith—these are the things I need the most right now. I am a wife and a mother, but in so many ways, I am still a child. I need to grow up, and I need to do it quickly. The future of my babies, my family, my whole life depends upon it.

Joyce turns onto the road that leads to the interstate, which we'll take for the next hour and a half, until we reach home. I have to break the news to everyone. Joyce could tell Tom's dad,

Don, but I'll have to find a way to tell Tom. And Carter. I can't even imagine what to tell a four-year-old. The burden of it feels overwhelming.

On the interstate, we join the rush of cars and trucks speeding by anonymously, and I think, *I could be anyone. No one knows I am the mother of a baby with Down syndrome. I am a normal woman, riding along in this car.* The thought soothes me. I like the idea of being anonymous. It feels easy, free.

But, although the babies are already five days old, I still look pregnant. There is a bright red scar below the pouch of my round belly, and my breasts are filled with mother's milk. My mind might let go of my circumstances easily and quickly, but my body doesn't. I am tied to my babies and tied to motherhood, whether I like it or not. The thought occurs to me that if I were to get in a car accident and die in an instant, the paramedics who find me would know everything simply by looking at my body. I'm a woman who had recently given birth, I'm in a car with three car seats, and I'm lactating. But where are the babies?

When I was pregnant, people would see me waddling toward them and clear a path. Strangers would pat my belly and say, "Oh, my, that's going to be a big baby." I'd smile and hold up my fingers in a peace sign and say, "Two. It's two babies."

"Better you than me!" or "My God, I feel so sorry for you" or "Get them on a schedule right away" were the replies. A Native American man with a long silver braid down his back broke into a big smile and said, "Double blessings!"

He was the first of the *twin people*, my name for the men and women who were in love with the idea of twins. My friend Phyllis, a homeschooling mother of five who says things like "She's a blessing in shoes," confided to me that with each pregnancy, she'd prayed for twins. My friend Sarah, a chic, liberal Democrat and mother of two boys, told me, "As a little girl, I

always imagined myself the mother of twins, a boy and a girl."
My sister had two cribs, two layettes, two of everything in her
attic waiting for the day she and her husband began their family.
They were hoping for twins. And from my mother's mother, my
gram: "I finally have my twins now. The last dream of my life has
come true."

Joyce glances over at me from time to time, but I look away. I'm
not ready to talk yet. Out the window, the town of Missoula recedes, its broad streets giving way to lanes, then dirt roads. Soon
we are in the country, surrounded by lodgepole pines and pon-
derosas and Douglas firs. I roll down the window and let the
breeze blow into my open mouth, like I used to do when I was
a kid. Even this brings fresh tears—memories of my childhood,
of me playing mommy, only never once did I play mommy to a
special needs child. I want it all back. All that time, back to the
days when my biggest concern was how much longer until the
streetlamps came on, because that was when I'd have to quit playing and go home.

Home to me then was a split-level ranch house on a quiet cul-
de-sac in the suburbs of San Francisco. My dad was an executive
at a marketing-research company, and my mom was a teacher.
Now home to me is a house at the end of a twisty gravel road,
on a hilltop rising from a peninsula that juts into Flathead Lake,
the largest body of fresh water west of the Mississippi. On a map,
the peninsula looks like an arm curled to show off its biceps. Our
house is on top of the middle finger's knuckle. From our two big
picture windows, you can see a hundred miles across the lake—all
the way to the ski slopes cut into the Whitefish mountain range,
or past the Swan Mountains to Heaven's Peak, one of the highest
points in Glacier National Park, or closer in, to a tiny teardrop of
land called Bird Island, maintained by the University of Montana
as a waterfowl sanctuary. Earlier in the morning, I'd watched

seven kayaks paddle out to the island, the lake flat, the sky clear. From my vantage point, the kayaks looked like colorful confetti spilled across a bright blue tablecloth.

We live in a single-story two-bedroom house with weathered gray siding and a rust-colored roof. When we learned two babies were coming, one of the first things Tom said was "We'll have to put an addition on the house. We'll need more room." He said this with an air of resignation, because we didn't have the money for more babies, or more house. I reassured him babies don't take up much space, at least at first, and that a new coat of paint on the old bedroom would be fine.

Because it was the request of a terribly pregnant woman, or because it was simply cheaper, we replaced talk of the addition with talk of paint color. We decided on a functional, if bland, off-white. Tom would do the painting, as I needed to stay away from the fumes. Carter could help. We opened all the windows and set up box fans, and the two men in my life, big and small, worked on the room. I'd sneak in and scribble words on the walls yet to be painted, things like "happiness" and "laughter" and "love," Carter's eyes growing big because I was writing on the walls. "It's okay, honey," I said. "We'll cover it all up, but it will still be there, like a secret, or a wish. For good things, for all of us." Tom was reluctant at first, but he got into the spirit and added "music" and "books." Carter asked that we write "sunshine" and "chocolate milk."

I can barely stand to think about that time now. We chose all the wrong things. We should have written "good health" or "normal chromosomes" or "please, let everything be okay." I want to peel up the paint to get to the words hidden underneath, turn it all back, do it over. How foolish I was. I can't stand the thought of that happy afternoon, and all those silly hopes surrounding me on all four sides.

The news is two hours old. Avery is five days old. I am thirty-six years old. These are the numbers. My pregnancy was described with two medical terms: "high risk" and "advanced maternal age." The "high risk" was because it was a twin pregnancy, "advanced maternal age" because I was older than thirty-five. We discussed it with my doctor. Usually, she recommends an amniocentesis for women of advanced maternal age. But since I was carrying twins with separate amniotic sacs, we would need two amnios. Two amnios would be twice the risk to the health of the fetuses. She suggested that we proceed with all the other diagnostic tests, such as the triple screen and the high-resolution ultrasound, and if anything came up abnormal, we could then have the amnios to confirm or deny the results.

She was saying that because I was an older mom, my babies were at a higher risk for birth defects and genetic anomalies, but testing for them might cause my high-risk pregnancy to miscarry. The choice was up to us. All of the ultrasounds showed we had two healthy baby boys, hearts and hands and heads in the right proportions, the triple screen came back normal, and my blood glucose levels were fine, so we decided to forgo the amnios. The risks associated with the procedures were greater than the likelihood of discovering any difficulty; we played the odds. At the time I remember thinking I wouldn't care if there were a problem. I'd love any baby just as it was. But I didn't really think it would come to that.

When you have a healthy newborn, doctors and nurses could say to you, "We're sorry to tell you that your life is about to change in innumerable ways, both big and small. You will be sleep-deprived over an extended period of time, which might cause depression or, worse, dementia, you will suffer a financial blow, and your marriage will be strained," but they don't. They wish you well and tell you how lucky you are. When you have a child with a problem, the news is different.

It's a bleak picture.

I think of the stereotypes: the thick neck, the big tongue, and the wide, staring eyes. I think of adult diapers, health problems, and poverty. I'm sickened with fear, and devastated at the grief I think I've brought down upon us, that happy threesome who not long ago was painting words of hope and faith on the bedroom walls. I'm ashamed, and my shame disgusts me. And yet I think, *If I have these thoughts, won't others have them, too?* My heart breaks again and again, for who I am, and for what I have done.

I still have to tell Tom.


The long journey from the hospital ends at our doorstep. Joyce takes my arm and guides me up the steps, gently opening the door for me as if I were an invalid, which perhaps I am. I can hear Carter saying, "Mommy's home. Mommy's home," and this brings more tears. I feel so utterly incapable of handling this, my life. Tom pops his head around the hallway and says, "What's up?" and it's more than I can bear. I rush through the house into our bedroom.

"Is everything okay?" Tom asks Joyce.

"The babies are growing and gaining weight. But we got some news today," she says and hesitates. I can hear all of this from the bedroom, and I think, *Now. I have to do it now.* This is my chance to step into the shoes of an adult. I need to claim this. I need to own it. I have to tell my husband what has happened.

I step out into the hall and grab Tom's sleeve, pulling him into our bedroom. I sit down on the bed, our bed, and begin talking. I can see the summer light coming through the blinds so clearly, so sharply. I can hear the words coming out of my mouth, even as I watch the dust settle around us. The light shifts imperceptibly toward the west. Sundown. The comforter cover glows a color from my childhood, burnt sienna, and I wonder if Avery will ever own a box of crayons, will ever color with them, will ever be able to read the words "burnt sienna" on the side of a Crayola.

It begins now.

It begins with the words I tell my husband—words I would find myself saying over and over again in the coming days and weeks.

Avery has Down syndrome.

This is the beginning of our story.

# 2

## Slipping

I'm moving through the air feetfirst, soaking wet. Fluorescent lights whiz in and out of sight. There's so much water. We turn left, we turn right. We stop. It's a bright, rectangular room. Out of the corner of my eye, I think I see brilliant shapes and colors painted on the walls. A red elephant. A purple giraffe. But this makes no sense. Maybe it's only a dream.

Two large round lights are positioned over me, like giant eyeballs. Hands and arms appear and move me from the gurney to a tall bed. My stomach is a mountain in front of me. I'm rolled onto my side, pulled into a sitting position, and given a shot of anesthesia in my spine. I slump back down and slowly stretch out, away from the contractions, away from myself, becoming numb. A face appears: a woman, wisps of blond hair around her face, wrinkles in the corners of her eyes. "Tom isn't here yet. The babies are ready. The doctor is ready. The nurses are in place, the anesthesiologist. The neonatologist, his nurse." Her voice is kind and lilting. I could listen to it forever. Everyone is waiting, including me. I am waiting for the voice to say something more.

"Are you ready?" it asks.

"Oh," I say. I hadn't realized I was supposed to answer. I consider it: am I ready?

The babies. We're at thirty-three weeks. Thirty-seven is

considered term for twins. Four weeks shy of that. But is that the question here?

I'd woken in the early-morning darkness to a wet, warm feeling on my legs. My first, sleepy thought was that I'd lost control of my bladder. My second, fear-induced thought was that it was blood. I rolled out of bed and into the bathroom, where I quickly peeled off my pants. In the dull pale dawn I couldn't see any blood. I switched on the bathroom light; my clothes were wet but clear. I looked more closely: still no blood.

I sat on the edge of the bathtub and rubbed my belly. I knew what this was. My water broke with my first pregnancy, too, weeks past the due date. This time, it was weeks early.

I wrapped towels around myself and waddled back into the bedroom to wake Tom. "My water broke," I said, pulling him from one dream into another. My main concern, at that moment, was what to do with Carter. My friends had small children of their own to care for, and because the due date was still so far away, Tom and I were alone.

"Are you sure?" he asked.

"Yes." While he pulled on clothes, I called the ER and explained my situation. The nurse on the other end of the line told me to come in.

We tucked Carter, still sleeping, into his car seat and the three of us drove to the local hospital, where the on-call ob-gyn, who wasn't my regular doctor, examined the babies and me. The contractions had begun, waves of pain that left me stunned and groggy. She ordered an IV drip of magnesium sulfate to forestall labor, and gave me a shot of betamethasone to hasten the babies' lung development. "We're going to have to ship you," she said apologetically. Tom went home, intending to pack a bag and change Carter out of his pajamas. I was loaded into an ambulance for the seventy-five-mile trip to the nearest NICU.

I remember the first moment I suspected I was pregnant: my morning coffee tasted so repulsive to me that I gagged. I looked at the calendar, counting back the days. Could it be? And the test, an Answer: two unmistakable pink lines.

I'd been working part-time writing a newsletter for a local organization that provides support to adults with disabilities. My last task, to wrap up the current edition, was to interview Sandy B., a fifty-year-old woman with Down syndrome who lived in the neighboring town in a house her brothers had built. I met her there, where we had strawberry-kiwi yogurts and she showed me her crayon collection. She was a pixie of a woman, with short gray hair, and we spoke for about a half hour. When I stood to go, she reached over and hugged me, holding on for a long while, gently patting my back. I don't know how she knew I needed a hug, but I did. For the first time in weeks, I felt as if everything would be okay. I felt it so keenly that it brought tears, and I remember going out to my car, putting on my sunglasses, and letting loose—crying great, racking, nose-dripping sobs of relief.

There was the ultrasound that showed not one but two babies. High risk. Adjusting our plans and expectations, telling others that we were having twins: "I can't believe that word is going to be a part of the rest of my life," I'd told my friend Sarah. Tom and I decided I should quit my part-time work and focus on the pregnancy. I was put on a special high-protein diet prescribed by a prenatal nutritionist. Twice-monthly checkups; frequent ultrasounds. The new used car; the clean coat of paint on the bedroom wall. All the while, trying to imagine the unimaginable: two babies, at once.

"Are you ready?" asks the nurse with the kind eyes.

"Can we wait for Tom?" I ask.

She disappears, then reappears. "No more than half an hour."

"A half hour," I repeat, nodding. I can see a big circular clock high on the wall to my left. The hands move strangely; and still, Tom is not here. The giant round lights are switched on, and a blue tarp is spread over me. It's time.

As the surgery begins, the nurse talks to me, telling me what's happening. I can feel a tugging sensation, a pulling. It's not painful. Everyone is busy. I can see the bobbing of blue caps above the blue tarp. "That's the first baby," I hear her say, an echo of the doctor's words. "Beautiful." And then, "Here's the second baby. Beautiful." I hear, "Baby A, eight nine." I hear, "Baby B, eight nine." The Apgars. I lift my head up and peek over the divider. I see a flash of newborn skin, then another, nurses and doctors all in motion.

Tom and Carter meet me in recovery.

"I missed it all," Tom says.

"I'm sorry," I say. "It was all ready to go. It was time."

"It's okay," he says, bending over to kiss my forehead. "It's all going to be okay."

I'm nauseous from the anesthesia; I'm shaking and sweating, and I can't stop scratching my nose. It feels so good to scratch my nose—with my fingers, my nails. Tom reaches out and grabs my hand. "Stop," he says gently. "It's getting really red."

I nod, then try to rub my nose against my shoulder, my arm.

"Stop," he says again.

"It's really itchy," I say, by way of explanation.

A nurse comes in and checks my pupils, takes my blood pressure, asks me how I'm feeling. I don't know the answer; what seems to be the closest word to what I'm feeling is "disappointment." It happened so fast—I arrived at the hospital, and the babies were delivered in less than an hour. On a normal day, I can't make it in and out of the grocery store that fast. But this isn't what she's asking me: it's a medical question. "My nose itches," I say.

"That's from the anesthesia," she explains. "It'll wear off."

Carter, Tom, and I are moved into a regular hospital room, and Tom begins making phone calls. Everyone is surprised; there was no warning. A nurse turns the television to Nick Jr., and Carter watches a show about a sponge boy who lives in a pineapple under the sea. The whole idea seems improbable to me, but then, so does my life. Carter giggles and belly laughs, so clearly life in a pineapple is a jolly one. The nurse also gives him both halves of an orange Popsicle and a paper cup to catch the spills.

The itching in my nose is subsiding, and the shakes are gone. I don't feel the euphoria I remember with Carter's birth. What is settling in around me, like a low fog creeping into the room underneath the doorway, is fear. I don't know what it means to have delivered these babies at thirty-three weeks.

When Carter was born, I saw them clean him. I watched as the nurse put a tiny diaper on him, and tucked his bald head into a little white cap. She bundled him in a blue blanket, and he was returned to me. I held him for the rest of the night. Sometime in the early morning, one of the night nurses wheeled his little plastic crib out of the room so I could rest; I woke immediately, got myself out of bed, and trudged out into the hall after her, to retrieve him. We were never apart.

I haven't held the twins.

I've barely even seen them.

I hold on, instead, to the Apgar scores, which I heard distinctly. Eights and nines. Eights and nines means that everything must be okay.


The hospital is quiet and dim. Because it's graduation weekend in this university town, there are no hotel rooms available, so Tom has taken Carter home to sleep. Two nurses help me into a wheelchair and push me down the wide corridor. One steps ahead and punches numbers into a keypad. The metal door pops open, and I'm wheeled past a tangle of machines, monitors, and other babies, to mine. Two little wrinkled boys, naked except for tiny diapers. Each is in a Plexiglas box. Each little chest is dotted with electrodes attached to wires leading to machines. Tubes taped into their nostrils. IV lines dripping a yellow solution into their bodies. A clamp stuck on each big toe, with a wire connected to a machine.

We had talked weeks of gestation like they were numbers at a garage sale—*Forty. No, thirty-six. Would you take thirty-four? Yes, to thirty-four, but not thirty-three. Thirty-three will get you shipped....You really need to give it thirty-four. Thirty-five would be better.*

I take it all in with a sinking feeling. It's the middle of the night; Tom has gone home with Carter. I am on my own, alone with the weight of it.

I begin to cry. They are too small. *No*, I think, *no. This is not right*. I want, with all my heart, to still be pregnant with these babies.

A cheerful nurse, yet another woman named Jennifer, asks me, "Would you like to hold them?"

I'm unsure. Would it hurt them? I seem unnecessary, superfluous, nothing more than a tired woman with a red nose. But I do want to hold them. I want to tuck them under my chin, feel them with me, a triangle of heartbeats as we had been just a half day before.

I nod yes.

Jennifer positions my wheelchair, then hands me the babies—Avery, Bennett. She disappears and returns with a digital camera. She takes a picture of me and my clown nose and my two tiny, wired babies. I try to manage a smile. There is one other mother in the NICU, a pregnant woman taking a tour. She's going to have a C-section because of preeclampsia. Her baby is at twenty-seven-weeks gestation. She's watching me, watching us.

"It's scary," she says.

"Yes," I say, because it is.

When I return to my room, there is a tray with tea and red Jell-O by my bed. There's also a little business card with a picture of a lake mostly hidden in fog, and the words *May my thoughts this day turn toward gratitude for all the gifts I have received,* printed in white script across the gray mist. I flip the card over and it reads, *For more information about Pastoral Care Services at CMC, call the Chaplain's office at 4063 or ask your nurse to contact the Chaplain for you.*

The little card bugs me. Did someone think I needed help? Who chose this particular card? Who's telling me I'm supposed to be grateful? And then I consider it. I think about Carter, and Tom, and home. I remember our friends and families, pulling for us. And two new lives, barely babies, sleeping quietly. My anger dissipates, leaving me feeling cleaned out, stripped bare of almost every emotion, save one: love. The only thing left is love for my boys, at home and down the hall.

When I was a new mother to Carter, electric breast pumps seemed creepy. Instead, I used a little Avent hand pump, which was as gentle and discreet as it was promised to be. It had plastic bottles that matched the pump, which matched the lids, and rims, and nipples. It was a tidy system and I embraced it.

But it's become clear to me that my trusty little Avent is the equivalent of trying to cut a two-acre lawn with a hand mower. While hand mowers are old-fashioned, and peaceful, and might be delightful on a sunny summer afternoon, a person in my situation has no time for quaint. Enter the heavy-duty equipment: the bright blue Medela Lactina Electric Plus with adjustable vacuum and speed, on loan from the hospital.

A nurse is showing me how to pour the milk from the two collection cups into plastic bags, two ounces each. Fold the top over and over, seal it with masking tape (Scotch tape is unreliable), mark the day and the time on the side with a black Sharpie, then affix a preprinted label with the boys' names and patient numbers.

We deliver the milk to a mini-refrigerator in the back of the NICU, where each mother has her own section. Mine is the left corner of the top shelf. Some of the other plastic Baggies in the fridge are slight, like mine; others are big hulking things filled to the brim. I begin to worry that my milk supply is inadequate, especially for twins.

The reality of having two premature babies is still fresh, and it seeps into my thoughts when I'm not expecting it. One minute I'm remembering when the breast pump was wheeled into my room, and I was studiously attaching the hoses and cups and bottles I'd purchased from the hospital (things that needed to be new to be sanitary), when Tom grabbed the collection cups and started speaking into them like they were microphones: "Testing, one, two, three." First one, then the other: "Check, check, testing, check." And the next minute, I'm thinking about the babies in their little plastic boxes, tubes and wires snaking around them.

I tell the nurse, who is my guide, that I'm tired and would like to go back to my room and wait for Tom.

It's a rainy afternoon and the hospital is quiet. My window looks out on a narrow alley. Every now and then the sun breaks through the clouds, illuminating the soft terra-cotta bricks of the building across from me, turning the vine growing up its side a bright, glowing green. I feel a fluttering in my stomach, and for a moment I think it's the babies moving. Then I realize it's just me—no more wiggles, no more babies. The sunshine recedes and the alley turns to mist again.

I go home in three days, but the babies? It's a question that inspires slippery answers. Sometimes I'm told, "It all depends," which leaves hope that they will come home with me. Other times, I hear, "A week, maybe ten days." Once: "Until they would have been term," meaning four weeks, maybe seven, depending upon which definition of "term" you use—term for twins, or term for a singleton pregnancy?

I vaguely remember a high school science class that involved discarding the highest value and the lowest value in a series, and I employ this technique here. I disregard the four-to-seven-week estimate—pretend as if it doesn't count—because I can't bear the thought of it; in fairness, I also give up the optimistic idea of the babies coming home with me, as if by striking this bargain, I'll have some say in how it turns out.

When Tom arrives, we hold hands on our way to the NICU. At the locked door, I speak into the air. "We're the parents?" I say. "Can we hold the babies?"

The door buzzes open and a nurse comes around the corner.

"Sure. Let me get you set up," she says.

She leaves for a moment and returns with warm blankets, which she hands to Tom and me and motions for us to follow her. She pulls over a wooden rocking chair painted pink, with a blue cushion on the seat, for me to use, and she offers Tom her swiveling office chair. We scoot in close to the isolettes.

Inside, each baby, naked except for a tiny diaper and a knit cap, is sleeping on a sheepskin, on his tummy, with little white blankets rolled tight on either side to position him—all things that are unfamiliar to me as a mother. I'd been taught that sheepskins were dangerous because babies might suffocate in them, that babies should sleep on their backs, and that cribs should be free of all bedding and blankets, even crib bumpers.

"Is this okay?" I ask.

"Different rules here," the nurse says. "We don't worry about SIDS with all this," she says and nods to the bank of monitors.

Each baby is connected to a machine that reminds me of the fish finder on Tom's dad's boat—three squiggly gray lines running across a green background. The pulse-ox keeps track of the blood oxygen content through a sensor clamped onto a big toe. A wired patch on each chest monitors heart rate, and another measures respiration rate.

Each baby has a tube taped to his mouth, for my breast milk, which they haven't begun receiving yet. Instead, they are being fed a yellow electrolyte solution through an IV, held in place with white tape winding around and around tiny arms.

The nurse opens the first isolette and gently lifts Avery, handing him to me. He has on a little purple-and-white knit cap. Next is Bennett, to Tom. His little cap is green and yellow, and it slides down over one side, giving him a jaunty look.

The fish-finder machine shows Avery's respiratory rate is zero.

"Um, is this all right here?" I ask nervously. The nurse leans over and resets the monitor.

"Sure," she says. "These things go off all the time. Look at the baby, if you're unsure. He's not blue or anything."

A little shudder goes through me at the thought of my baby turning blue, and I wonder if I will ever get used to this place, where such things are part of ordinary conversation.

Bennett's monitor goes off next—he has kicked off his toe clamp. It's an insistent beeping that puts me on edge. I feel shaky and timid, like a skittish cat. Tom is uncomfortable, too. He's tapping the heels of his boots quickly and sharply against the linoleum floor. The nurse resets Bennett's monitor, and helps us switch babies. The pulse-ox goes off a second time, and the nurse resets Bennett's toe clamp. Our presence seems to cause trouble. Aside from dropping off the milk, I'm unsure of what else I'm supposed to do.

If you ask the same question twice in the NICU, you will get two different answers. But if you ask it often enough, eventually you will get a consensus, and that's as good as it's going to get. For instance, I ask why I can't hold the babies longer. One answer is "It's the rules." Another answer: "You can't hold them at all. You can only breast-feed them." Another: "You can hold them all day, if you want." But most often, I'm told it's because being in the "outside air" puts stress on their systems, and they need to grow, and the best place for them to grow is in their isolettes. I accept this as fact.

I've also come to believe the night nurses are nicer, and more apt to tell me things. The NICU at night is quiet, and there are fewer people around, so it seems as if everything is less rushed. The nurses have time to explain to me what each machine does, why it's important, and how it helps the babies, which helps me become less anxious.

Like all organizations, the NICU has a hierarchy. The nurses who watched over the babies and me the first night were the most experienced ones. When we had settled, and it was clear that we were well on our way, they were reassigned to babies with more difficult conditions.

The babies who are "feeders and growers," as I learned ours were called, are moved toward the front, where it's busier. The babies with the biggest challenges are kept in the back, where it's private and quiet. When I'd drop off my milk in the refrigerator, which was also in the back, I'd peek at the babies there. The isolettes were covered in quilts, and each baby had its own nurse, always nearby.

This is what I learned about NICU nurses: many have personal ties to premature babies. Some have mothered their own preemies; others have lost a baby prematurely. Sometimes I'd hear them whispering to the babies; once I saw a nurse kissing the top of a knit cap. I don't know how they can love them the way they do, and then say good-bye.

It's early morning in the NICU. I'm in my flimsy hospital gown, and my hair is pulled back into a ponytail. Our doctor, Jennifer, has been nothing but kind and professional. Each time something new develops, she tells me of it, and tries to explain it in a way that I'll understand. I trust her; better still, I like her. So when she comes over to me while I'm with the babies, and tells me that she wants to run some genetic tests on Avery, at first I don't understand the importance of it.

"Okay," I say. "What sort of tests?"

"There's a crease in his palm, and his ears are a little low on his head," she says.

"Great," I say, still not getting it. I begin folding up the blankets—a yellow one, then a blue striped one.

"I'm concerned that he might have Down syndrome," she says.

I stop. I look at her.

"It's going to be okay," she says. "I just want to check."

I wait for her to say more. She waits for me to ask a question. The air hangs heavy between us. Finally, she nods and walks away.

I'm still holding the blue striped blanket, which I twist around my hand. I can't think straight. I don't want to cry here. I mumble something to anyone, and no one, about going to my room. Before I know it, I am there. On the tray table beside my bed are a cup of tea and another little card. I pick it up. It's a lake at sunset, with words printed across the sky in black italics: *Courage is not the absence of fear, but the affirmation of life despite fear.*

Courage? Now courage? It's too much—I begin to cry. Who is sending me these messages that seem like handpicked responses to the most current crisis in my life? All my frustration, all my anxiety narrows to a single point of determination—I must know where these cards are coming from.

I rush out of my room and begin walking down the hall, sobbing. I pass an open doorway on my right and look inside. No tray, no cards. Ahead. On my left, another room. I look inside. No tray, no card. I keep walking. In my left hand is the card from the tray in my room; my right hand is holding the blue baby blanket wrapped around my fist as if I were wounded. Occasionally, I lift the blanket and wipe the tears from my face with it. The hallway takes a turn. I follow it. Coming toward me is Doc Hollywood.

"Are you okay?" he asks, concerned. I'm in my hospital gown, puffy-eyed from crying, going from room to room. "Are you lost?" he asks.

I wave the card at him, and begin to try to explain—to say it so that it will make sense—and realize that it doesn't make any sense at all.

"They want to test Avery for Down syndrome," I manage, and let out a loud, hiccuping sob.

"And you just found this out?" he asks.

"Yes."

He is a big man, tall like my father. He says nothing for a moment; then he reaches out and pulls me into a great bear hug. "I lifted him out of you," he says. "I didn't see anything wrong. It's okay." He releases me from the hug. "It's going to be okay."

A nurse has joined us, and each of them takes an arm, guiding me back to my room. The tray is gone, the tea is gone, and all that's left is the card that I hold in my hand. I tuck it into my journal, with the first one. When Tom comes a short while later, I tell him about the test, and we decide not to mention it to anyone else.

We agree that it's nothing.


By my fourth day in the hospital, the only thing that's clear is that the babies aren't coming home with me. I'd tried to arrange to room in, but the hospital is too full. I'd considered getting a hotel, but rooms are still hard to find and are very expensive. The only thing to do is go home and commute, but leaving without the babies feels like a failure.

As I'm packing up my things—rolling my fleece socks into a ball, gathering up the pens and notebooks and children's books I'd read to Carter—a woman comes into my room holding a tray from the cafeteria. She is short and middle-aged, and she has a long, pointy nose. She's dressed in a uniform of brown trousers, a brown shirt, and a white smock. Her hair is in a plastic shower cap. She's wearing plastic gloves. The brownness, and her long nose, and her plastic hat, remind me of Mrs. Tiggy-Winkle, the hedgehog from *The Tale of Mrs. Tiggy-Winkle and Mr. Jeremy Fisher*. She nods, and holds out the tray. I'm supposed to take it.

I scan its contents. A plate covered with a stainless steel dome, a carton of chocolate milk, a cup of tea, and another little card.

"Did you bring me these?" I ask.

She smiles at me. She has a crooked front tooth. I'm not sure that she understands. I try again. "Where did you get these cards?" I ask, taking out the other two and fanning them on the bed.

She smiles again, and nods. Maybe she doesn't speak English. It's not clear what I'm really trying to ask her, anyway. I abandon my interrogation, feeling foolish. I don't know what I was expecting to find—certainly not this, a small woman who may or may not be a character from a Beatrix Potter book.

She nods at me again, as if asking permission to leave.

"Thank you," I say, taking the tray from her.

"Thank you!" she repeats, backing out of the room.

I peek under the stainless steel dome—beef stroganoff, a wheat roll, green beans. I lift the little card, this one a picture of a lush green forest with the words *The Lord is my shepherd; I shall not want. In green pastures you give me repose; beside still waters you lead me; you refresh my soul.* I lay it on the bed with the other two, not sure what to do with them. I'd half convinced myself they had supernatural powers, my very own *woo-woo cards*. Now that I'm leaving, I'm on my own.

At home, Joyce has made a Welcome Home feast of meat loaf and mashed potatoes, and for dessert, a special treat—huckleberry pie. I try to be festive, try to be happy, and part of me is happy to be home, but another part is sick that the babies aren't with me.

I can't let it go. I'd wanted to make it to thirty-six weeks, at least. I'd wanted the babies to be born in the birthing room I'd toured at the local hospital, with the big windows that looked out over the town, across the lake and to the mountains in the east. I'd had it all planned out in my head—how I'd watch the sunrise from my hospital bed, how the babies would be nearby, how the three of us could look across the lake to the peninsula of land where, in the middle, on the top knuckle of the fist, sits our home.

I feel broken and fragile, unsteady and suspicious, as if everything might fall apart at any minute. After dinner, Joyce tells me to relax, but I can't. I begin cleaning out the refrigerator, throwing out my pregnancy food—the soy protein powder and the flaxseed oil and the CLIF Bars and the wheatgrass juice. The expiration date on a carton of yogurt brings tears to my eyes—it's the date the babies were supposed to be born. I toss it out, and ask Tom to take the plastic garbage bag away.

When I finish, I take Carter into his bedroom, and instead of reading him a bedtime story, I tell him a story about his brothers. I tell him babies come into the world in all kinds of ways, and our babies came early, so we have a whole team of people helping them and helping us. I say the hospital is like one giant crib for the babies to live in, and the nurses and doctors are all mommies and daddies looking out for them until they are bigger and stronger. I tell him they'll never be lonely, and never be sad, and we'll be with them a little while each day until they can come home with us forever.

On the surface, Carter seems to be taking me at my word.

And yet I wonder—the relaxed rules, all the sodas and candy, Grandma and Grandpa at his beck and call—he must realize something is not right.

The full moon hangs over the Mission Mountains, which I can see from our window in the family room. There is snow on the highest peaks and the moonlight turns them milky blue. It's midnight and the house is quiet except for the *whhshh-shshhh, whhshhh-shhh* of the electric breast pump. It's all about the milk.

I pump every three hours, though the lactation nurse tells me I should pump every two. The day for me, pumping every three, is divided into eight sections—six at home, two at the hospital. I can fit my life in around these sections. If I were to follow the lactation nurse's advice, my life would be split into twelve sections. I can't manage my life—spending time with Carter, driving to and from the hospital, visiting the babies, seeing Tom, occasionally sleeping—in two-hour segments. While pumping more often might be "optimal for milk production," I don't think the lactation nurse is keeping the big picture in mind. She's a chipper woman with short blond hair in a sweeping pageboy. She wants me to know she is a mom, she's been there, and she knows it's hard but it's what's best for the *babies*. I agree; my issue is with the fact that the babies are not the only ones with an interest in the situation. I have to think of what's best for the *family*.

I finish my little chore, and still, I can't sleep.

Worry over the genetic test is always there in the background, like a buzzing in your head that you simply endure, hoping it will go away soon. Until you find out the results. Then you wish you'd waited a little longer—you wish you'd had just a little more time. Another week, even, living the life you thought you had, believing in it, until the moment everything changes.

There is the summer light coming through the slats in the blinds. There is the comforter the color of a brown crayon. There is Tom, looking at me, his eyes intent, full of fear. He knows something is wrong. It's cruel to make him wait while I try to find the right way to tell him. So I say it, plain and bare.

"Avery has Down syndrome."

He doesn't say anything, but instead turns away from me so I can't see his face, but I can tell from the way his shoulders rise and fall that he has begun to cry.

I want to reach out to him, to hold him, to tell him that this is nothing, that this news is simply a bump in life, and everything will be okay. I want to tell him I love him, our love is bigger than this trouble; it's big enough to absorb all of it and more, if need be. But I say nothing, because I'm not sure I believe it myself. I begin crying, too, more tears, and I think, *How much?* How many tears can a person shed before they finally run dry?

Tears, his and mine, separate. My love for Tom is the finest thing I've known, the greatest experience in my life, and I might be losing it. It's what I'd most dreaded—that something, or someone, would break us, pull us apart from each other. I had thought it would be death. This is a death of sorts, perhaps. It feels final and irrevocable, hopeless, helpless.

It's hard to know what Tom is thinking.

Tom's shoulders are still heaving; he is not looking at me.

"I have to tell you something else, too," I begin. "One of the nurses told me there are families who adopt babies with Down syndrome."

I stop, leaving the idea hanging out there in the slanted sunlight, the dusty air. It's an ugly thought. That a baby of mine, of my body, of me, is the subject of it sickens me. But like all the news I bring home from the NICU, I don't filter it. I report it so that Tom can make up his own mind. I feel I owe him the truth, as best as I can relay it.

If he were to tell me, *Yes, go ahead, sign the papers,* I'd have to choose. My mind flashes to Carter, his four-year-old body, the sweet smell of his hair. Carter and Tom on one side, and a little wrinkled baby in a Plexiglas box miles and miles away from me on the other. The pain again becomes physical. It's an impossible scenario.

Tom stops me. "No," he says quietly, "no." Then he says again, "No. We won't do that." He turns and pulls me into a great, awkward hug, and I catch my breath and choke a little, but I can feel myself almost smiling. The worst thing is not happening. We will go forward, and though I can't see the way yet, we will find it together.

We stay like this for a while, holding on to each other, and then Tom pats me and releases me. Something has occurred to him.

"My dad," he says. "Does my dad know?"

"I'm not sure. Maybe your mom told him," I say.

"I should talk to him."

"Let me," I offer. "You sit awhile. I'll talk to him."

"No. I'll do it. It should be me. I should be the one."

He gets up and walks through the bedroom door, through the house and out onto the porch, where Don is cooking Johnsonville brats on the gas grill, his back to us, the dappled sunlight coming through the Douglas fir trees, a gentle breeze coming off the lake. He is wearing khaki shorts, white ankle socks, and a teal green golf shirt.

The sausages are steaming in a tin pan of beer, Don's tried-and-true method. When the beer has evaporated, the sausages go on the fire to brown and then they're done. It's an ordinary summer scene, played out over and over again across the country, families barbecuing to their exact special recipes, and I am overwhelmingly grateful for it, this familiar sight, that now seems to me so beautiful and sad. I love Don for cooking the bratwurst just so.

"Dad," Tom says, placing his hands in his pockets and looking down at his feet. He is wearing leather lace-up cowboy boots, Wranglers, and a long-sleeved button-down shirt. Don turns to face us.

"They did some tests on Avery and, well, we got the results back today." Tom shifts his weight from one foot to another, then takes his hands out of his pockets. He reaches over to me and grabs my hand and begins swinging it back and forth, a nervous gesture that makes me think of the last time I remember him doing it, which was on the shores of this same lake, on a sunny June morning almost exactly eleven years ago, our wedding day. It's the only sign of how hard this is for him.

Tom continues swinging and says, "It looks like Avery has Down syndrome."

Don doesn't hesitate. He hugs Tom, then hugs me, then says, "Ahhh, well, shoot."

He hugs me again, then Tom, and he steps back, leaving his hand on Tom's shoulder, a protective fatherly gesture. Tom leans into the arm, and looks down at his feet. I have seen them like this a hundred times. Don, the father, Tom, the son, connected by that touch. Sometimes, Don will reach over and adjust the back of Tom's collar, or smooth the shoulders of his shirt. In those moments, I can see back in time to the little boy Tom was, and Don as he was, a man about Tom's age now. It is clear to me that your children are always your children, despite all the growing up.

The beer has evaporated from the tin pan, so Don puts the sausages on the grill to brown. Whatever grief he may be feeling for himself, for his child, for the child of his child, he sets aside.

"About ten minutes left out here," he says quietly, helping us try to resume our lives. It's my cue to go into the house and tell Joyce supper is almost ready, and then we will set the table, and Carter will put the napkins out, counting, "One, two, three, four, five," in his careful and serious way.

I'm so thankful for these small familiarities. They are my guideposts in a day that has turned over and over on itself so many times, a day that has had all the qualities of a nightmare or a daydream, a day that has been full of equal parts despair and hope. I walk into the kitchen and give the ten-minute warning, suddenly as starving as a woman recently returned from the dead.

# 3

## Please, Come Back to Me

The next morning dawns bright, and I wake feeling as if I drank too much red wine the night before. The sunlight hurts my eyes and my skin feels stretched too tightly across my face. I'm up before everyone else to pump milk, and as I sit and try to think pleasant, happy thoughts so the milk will come, I begin crying again. I'm remembering a man at the thrift store in a nearby town. He has a wide oval face, soft sloping shoulders, and a great pouch of a belly. Every time we go into the store, he announces to me that it's his birthday. Can he have a hug? I always oblige, embracing him stiffly and quickly.

It makes Tom mad and sometimes we fight over it. "It can't be his birthday *every* day," he argues. "You're just indulging him." Whenever he sees the man coming over to me, he pulls Carter a little closer and goes to the other side of the store.

What's upsetting me now is this man's mother—I'd never once considered her. It never occurred to me that somewhere there is a woman who held him as a little baby, who changed his diapers, who rocked him and sang to him and cradled him through the night. I never considered the baby, the child, the family. In my mind, it was as if the man had always been grown, had always lived in the thrift store, waiting to tell me each month that it's his birthday. By denying him a childhood, I'd made him less than a full person. And now I wished I knew about it. How did he get there? Where is his family? Where is his mother?

Of course there is hardly any milk in the collection cups. Crying is not good for milk production. I finish and pack the milk in my little blue insulated cooler. I rinse out the shields and the bottles and put them in their little plastic bag, to take with me to the hospital. Carter is awake, Don and Joyce and Tom, too, and we all eat breakfast around the big table. Joyce has made eggs and toast for Carter, juice in a sippy cup. The table faces a window that looks out across the lake, which is a deep, rich blue, dazzling in the morning sunlight.

We decide to all make the trip to the hospital. It seems right for the whole family to arrive together as a team, Avery's team. We walk through the automatic revolving door, Don and Tom first, Joyce second, Carter and me last, holding hands.

Inside, the air is cool and artificially sweet. It smells like sickness and trouble covered up with flowers, Sterisoap, and hospital detergent. We deposit ourselves in one of the booths in the gift shop, surrounded by Mylar balloons with cheery sentiments like *Get well soon!* or *Feel Better!* or *It's a Girl!* and *It's a Boy!* There are some tired-looking roses in a glass-fronted refrigerator, and a rack of cards. One wall is devoted to snacks and has three vending machines—one for frozen treats, one with cookies and candies, one with soda and bottled water. To the left of the snack wall, there is an espresso bar doing a brisk business. The machine's screeching and sputtering grates on my overly raw nerves. It sounds like screaming.

Tom and I leave Carter with Don and Joyce and head to the NICU. To get there, we walk down the wide windowless corridor, the same corridor I was wheeled down on a gurney six days earlier. We are each wearing hospital ID wristbands, which we raise to show the nurse, who buzzes us into the NICU.

Inside the locked door, to the right, there are a sink and a pump bottle of Sterisoap. To the left, there are a little room with a chair and an ancient breast pump, for mothers to use while they are here. The room is the size of a closet and cluttered with old thumbed copies of *Parents* and *BabyTalk* and *People*, so well read the pages are soft as cloth. On the wall is a poem called "Tiny Feet," about big things growing from small beginnings. I know the poem is meant to be uplifting, but right now it seems impossible to imagine, like thinking of an oak tree while holding an acorn in the palm of your hand. I might be able to imagine the acorn sprouting; if I try, I can imagine a sapling. What lies beyond feels like too much to hope for. A laminated sign hanging from the door reads, THE BREASTFEEDING ROOM IS and then IN USE or FREE. Right now it reads, FREE.

Tom takes off his baseball cap and sets it on the ground near the door to the Breastfeeding Room, then begins washing his hands at the sink, one thousand one, one thousand two, one thousand three, one thousand four, one thousand five, as the nurses had shown us. I take off my coat and put it near Tom's hat, set down my little cooler, then begin to wash, too. Next to the sink there is a stack of clean hospital gowns. We each take one and put it on over our street clothes. I retrieve my cooler and go into the Breastfeeding Room, to pump and think about the poem and read old magazines.

Fifteen minutes later I emerge and take my bottles and my insulated cooler to the little fridge in the back. Tom is already with the babies. They are in the front, their little isolettes covered with patchwork quilts, their little bodies positioned so their eyes can look at black-and-white images meant to stimulate vision. Only when I get there, I see Avery's has been removed.

"Why is Avery's developmental thingy gone?" I whisper to Tom.

"I don't know."

"Maybe it fell down." We make a quick search of the isolette, the floor around the babies, the papers near them. Nothing.

"Bennett has two," Tom says. "Take one of his."

I do. Just as I am taping it to Avery's isolette, a nurse comes over.

"Can I help you?" she asks. She's a new nurse, one I don't recognize. She has on the royal blue scrubs of the NICU and has a stethoscope looped around her neck. On the desk next to the IV stand, there is a half-eaten bagel with cream cheese and a plastic container of orange juice.

Our section has three babies in it—our two, plus the twenty-seven-weeks gestation baby. I want to ask after him, and his mother, the woman who was on the little tour the first time I held the babies. But I don't. It's not allowed. If you ask about the other babies, or their families, the nurses turn stony and tell you it's confidential. I know this policy is supposed to protect the babies, and us, but it makes me feel lonely. We're all in this together, and yet we can't even know each other's names. I decide to think of the twenty-seven-weeks-old baby as Owen. Avery, Bennett, and their first friend, Owen.

Avery needs another test. His last blood culture showed bacteria, which might mean he has an infection. I hold Bennett, while the new nurse takes Avery from Tom and puts him back in his isolette. Sunshine is streaming in through the skylight. Avery begins crying, fussing. The nurse works over him. She tries to get a "good stick," but his veins are so small. Avery's crying grows louder, and Bennett, still on my chest, lifts his head and cries.

"A sympathy cry," the nurse says.

I feel like crying, too. I ask her if when the blood draw is done, I can hold them both. We carefully arrange each next to the other on my chest. I breathe them in, kiss their soft, fuzzy heads. They don't smell like Tom or me or Carter, or like baby lotion, or like milk. They smell like the NICU.

It's over too quickly. Time to put them back, time to let them rest. I go back to the Breastfeeding Room to pump again. When I return, the nurse makes marks on a huge spreadsheet at her desk, then gets up to see us out. We are the visitors; she is the host.

She's carrying a thick white binder. I think it's more paperwork, but as she follows us out, she says, "Here, this is for you. Some of us nurses thought you should have it."

I take it from her, unsure of what it might be. There is a paper in the clear front of the binder that reads, *We're U.P. @ The Down Syndrome Connection.* It continues, *Our children are a gift, a blessing and our heritage! Especially for you from parents in Missoula MT and surrounding area.* I don't know what to say. I hadn't realized the news would have spread, though of course I should have assumed it. Then I remembered Avery's isolette.

"Could you do me a favor?" I ask. "Could you make sure Avery's black and white image stays in his isolette? When we got here this morning, it was gone."

"Sure," she says. "I'll make a note of it."

Carter's small hand is in mine as we step off the curb into the parking lot. As short as our visits are, it's all I can manage. Any more time inside, and I begin to feel as if I'm suffocating; any less time, and my body begins to ache for the babies. I am running up and down a seesaw; as soon as one end gets too high, I turn and rush to the other: up and down, back and forth across the miles. The five of us pile into the Expedition—Don and Tom in front; Joyce, Carter, and me in the middle. The third-row backseat is empty.

We have lunch at Fuddrucker's, a loud, crowded, noisy restaurant where I always eat too much and feel slightly ill afterward, but it's a kid-friendly place. Carter gets a red balloon and soda in a red-and-white go-cup, and he is delighted. Without actually speaking about it, we are all feeling protective of Carter, trying to shield him from the worst of it, trying to pretend as if this is all just a part of life, babies in the hospital and mommies with red-rimmed eyes.

Carter calls Missoula "Busytown" after a place in a Richard Scarry book. Missoula's four-lane highways, its strip malls and shopping centers, the university and the airport make it a busier place than our hometown. We make one stop before leaving Busytown, to a bookstore.

Books are our lifeblood—they introduced me to Tom, and they probably convinced Tom to move west, though he denies it. I had my first crush on a boy simply because he loved reading as much as I did. My second crush was on Tom, who loved books even more than I did. I went to college to try to learn to write them, and in college I met Tom, who had the same plan. He graduated a year ahead of me and moved to Colorado, to work on a dude ranch high in the Rocky Mountain town of Breckenridge. Our letters to each other were our first collaboration; three years later we were married in front of family and friends on the shores of Flathead Lake, which seems both like yesterday and a very long time ago.

We stop in the bookstore because Tom's first book is out, and he wants to find it and hold it in his hands. Crack it open to the smell of fresh ink, and see the pages and pages of his words transformed. I remember the first time I touched a book with my name in it; I opened the stiff new binding to my essay, and tears came to my eyes. There was a man standing next to me looking at another copy, and I wanted to hug him, and tell him life is wonderful, and maybe point out my name to him and say, "See? That's me!" But of course I didn't. Instead I tried to act nonchalant, like it was no big deal to be weeping over a stack of anthologies.

We find Tom's book, and it is beautiful, sitting there on the shelf face out for all the reading world to see. I'm watching Tom, and he seems distracted. Finally, he leaves the aisle. I can only guess what he's thinking, with so many big things happening at the same time. Maybe it's all too much.

Usually, a bookstore is my favorite place to be. But I'm not feeling like myself. I'm not interested in looking at the new releases. Bargain books don't tempt me. Now that we've left the NICU, all I want to do is get home so I can call the nurses and find out if anything has happened since we left. Joyce and I take Carter to the children's section, and Don wanders down the history aisle. After a while, we all amble toward the checkout.

Tom meets us there. He has a book in his hands, which he gives to me. *Babies with Down Syndrome: A New Parents' Guide*, edited by Karen Stray-Gundersen. *The first book that parents and family should read,* it says on the cover. Tom shrugs his shoulders. "What do you think?" he says.

I'm happy and sad and surprised all at once. I should have known where he was going. Of course he would get a book, and it means many things to me: it means he's really "in" this whole deal; it means he's ready to begin trying to understand it; it means he is the same Tom he's always been.

"Sure," I say. "Let's get it." I add it to the books in my arms for Carter, *Blueberries for Sal* by Robert McCloskey (Mommy-sanctioned) and a book about Thomas the Tank Engine (Carter-sanctioned). Joyce has *The Red Tent* by Anita Diamant, which her book club will be discussing. Tom and Don go back and forth on who will pay, but Don takes out his credit card faster, and says, "Let me do this."

We all pile into the car again and begin the long drive home. Carter looks at his Thomas book, then falls asleep in his car seat. Don dozes in the front passenger seat. I'm sitting behind him. I watch Busytown recede, the streets giving way to lanes, giving way to dirt roads, then trees. We follow the highway as it rises up out of the little cup of the valley that holds our babies, up and up, and soon I can see the wall of the Mission Mountains rising in front of us, massive and solid. They seem close enough to touch.

I put my hand to the window as if to trace the craggy ridges, like a woman in the dark trying to find her way by feel, but there is only the smooth surface of the glass, and the hum of the car's air conditioner, which sounds for all the world like the HVAC we'd just left behind.

Soon enough we are home. We disentangle ourselves from the seat belts, the car seat. We gather up the bottles of water and the red-and-white go-cup, my little blue cooler (now empty), Ziploc Bags of pretzels and raisins, the new books. I head immediately into the house, note there are no new messages on the machine, and dial the number for the hospital, which I know by heart.

I ask after the babies. The nurse on the other end of the line seems to know who I am right away. "They're doing great!" she says in a chipper voice.

"Well, um, okay," I say. "We're home now, just wanted you to know. You can reach us here if you need anything." I feel silly for having disturbed her, for having added one more buzzing noise to the din of the beeping machines that I can hear in the background. We say good-bye and I hang up. I go back to our bedroom, to pump again.

When I'm done, I find that Carter and Grandpa have gone for a walk. A wander, or a meander, might be more accurate. Joyce and I discuss dinner options; we all had a big, late lunch, so we settle on the reheated turkey soup Joyce brought and salad. There are three sausages left from the night before, too. We fix things and put out plates, napkins. The clink of silverware, the smell of soup warming on the stove, these things calm me. It feels good to be home.

After supper I excuse myself again. I feel like the disappearing woman, every three hours slipping away from the ebb and flow of family life, hoping no one will notice, trying to be discreet. There isn't much milk, and I know I need to try harder to relax, and to eat, and to rest. I still have phone calls to make. I don't have any more information than I did yesterday, and nothing seems to be getting any easier or better. I briefly think of trying to convince Tom to call for me, but it doesn't feel right to hide from it. The responsibility is mine. There's an hour time difference, and if I wait too long, it will be too late.

I think of all the phone calls I've had to make to my parents over the years. Missed curfews. A car accident. The time I decided I wanted to take a year off from college. Moving west with Tom. The two of us deciding to build a life here, thousands of miles away. And still, they are nothing at all, compared to this. It will be the hardest call of my life.

I dial the numbers. I say the words over and over again: "Avery has Down syndrome, Avery has Down syndrome, Avery has Down syndrome," to my mom, to my dad and his wife, Pam, to my only sibling, Glynnis.

Dad says, "He'll be one of the better ones," and Pam says, "He's healthy, right? That's all that matters. He'll do great."

Mom says, "Oh, my," then, "Honey, is there anything I can do for you?"

Glynnis says, "I'm proud you are my sister."

It's a blur of tears and the words *I love you* and *It will be okay* and *Keep in touch* and it's done.

I have to concentrate to keep my hands from shaking.

I breathe. Inhale, exhale. There are still more people to call, but it will have to wait. For now I am done.

I pack up my things, take my milk cups and the phone back to the kitchen. I put the milk in the storage bags, two ounces each. I fold the tops over and over, tape them down with masking tape. I write on them, "6/14," then "6 p.m.," with a black Sharpie. I peel off a computer label from the sheet and affix it to the back. I stack the four little bags on the top shelf of the fridge. Finally, I mark a thick black X through the day on the calendar. As I look, I notice tomorrow is Father's Day.

We have a little house on a hilltop near a pretty lake. It's a house filled with books, made better with the how-to advice of books. There are words beneath the paint on the walls, words like "sunshine" and "happiness" and "chocolate milk."

It is a small house, two bedrooms and two baths. But it feels big, because of the many large windows that look out across the lake, and windows that face the deep bluing mass of the Mission Mountains. The sun rises over them each day, and some nights, the moon follows. Watching the full, bright disk as it lifts above the snowy peaks, climbing higher and fuller into the starry sky, is one of the very best reasons for living here, and a feature of the house the Realtor who showed it to us wasn't aware of.

His name was George, and he was hard of hearing at all the right times. When we told him our budget, or our requirements, he would say, "Hmmm? Could you speak up?" But when we whispered to each other that we were getting tired of looking at ugly places, his hearing would perk up and he'd say, "Ah, don't give up yet! I have one more place to show you! You're going to love it!"

It was exasperating. I was carrying six-month-old Carter around in a front pack, kangaroo-style. We'd bounce in and out of the car, in and out of other people's houses, each one a little more wrong than the last. We were ready to give up when Tom noticed a listing we hadn't seen.

"What about this?" he asked, pointing to the price.

"Oh, you wouldn't like that. It's too far from town and there's only two bedrooms."

"Still, is that the right price?" Tom asked.

"Let me check. Yes."

"Could we look at it?" I asked.

"I'll tell you what. I'll give you a map with directions, and you can drive out there on your own, and if you like it, you can call me and we'll go from there."

We took the map and drove alongside the base of the mountains, then turned west onto a twisty gravel road that led to the house. It was small and far from town, just as George had promised. But he didn't know about the two-and-a-half-car garage down the hill from the little house, with an attached workshop and office. It was more than enough space for us, back when we were a threesome.

When we learned we were having twins, we thought the babies would share a bedroom with Tom and me. Carter would keep his room, the only room he's ever known since we signed the closing papers on the house. In one corner is a twin bed with dragonfly sheets. There is a bench below the window, which looks out at the mountains. Across from the bed is an old dresser, painted dark blue and red. White walls, cream-colored carpeting, wood blinds, wood trim on the wood closet door, a bear with a parachute hanging from the ceiling. Toys litter the floor—tiny Matchbox cars, little toy trains, a wooden rocking horse, and books. *Harold and the Purple Crayon*, *Guess How Much I Love You*, *Goodnight Moon*. In the bed is a towheaded boy, asleep. I gently close the door.

Don and Joyce have gone down to the sofa bed in the office for the night, and the house is quiet. The dishwasher is going, and Tom has the radio playing softly. I can see him from across the room, sitting on our faded green couch, staring blankly out the window, now black with night. Tears are streaming down his cheeks. On the couch next to him is the new book, facedown like a little tent. I go to him.

"Are you okay?" I ask. He nods. I pick up the book and flip through the pages. Words like "Heart Defects" and "Leukemia" and "Life-Saving Surgery" jump out at me. There are more, in bold type and impossible to miss: Respiratory Problems, Gastrointestinal Problems, Vision, Hearing, Thyroid Problems, Orthopedic Problems, Dental Concerns, Seizures. My God, if this is "the first book that parents and family should read," what's the second?

I sit down beside him. "Are you really okay?" I put my arm on his back, and he turns his head to me.

"I was reading," he says. "It was going along fine. I kept thinking, 'Okay, I could handle that. Yeah, that would be okay.' And then I came to the part where it says, 'Babies with Down syndrome have mental retardation.' Boom. It was so definitive, so final. It took away any hope."

I don't know what to say. Because we are a family of books, we are likely to give them too much weight, too much importance. I'm suspicious of a book that could reduce Tom to tears. I thumb through it cautiously. I see black-and-white pictures of children, graphs, charts, forms. The chapters cover such topics as medical concerns and treatments, daily care of your new baby, family life, development, teaching your baby, and legal rights and hurdles. There's a glossary of terms in the back. I read some of the *A*s: abstractions, actuarial, ADA, adaptive behavior, adenoids, advocacy groups, alpha A-crystallin gene.

On the facing page, there are three short statements. I read them—accusations of people abusing the system, descriptions of children in institutions—then make myself stop, because I can't see how such comments are appropriate in a book for new parents. I don't know whose words they are—there's no name on any of the quotes in the "Parent Statements" section. I'm not ready for it. I put the book on the shelf and cover it with Louise Erdrich's *Love Medicine*, as if I could make the hurt go away. I kiss Tom on the forehead, and he goes to bed.

I don't follow him—instead, I open the binder from the hospital. The first page is a welcome letter, with words like "congratulations" and "triumph" and the phrase "beautiful new baby." The next page is titled "Welcome to Holland," by Emily Perl Kingsley. At the bottom, there is a black-and-white-and-gray photocopy of a picturesque Dutch scene—soft rolling hills and a little house topped with a windmill. I begin reading.

Emily Perl Kingsley is a mother of a son with Down syndrome. She's often asked to describe the experience, she explains, to help others imagine how it would feel. It's like this, she says: expecting a baby is like planning a fabulous trip. Everyone you know, including you, is planning to go to Italy. But after months of eager anticipation, you get the news that your arrangements have changed. You still go on a trip, but not to Italy. The place you're in isn't a bad place—it's just different. Slower-paced. Less flashy. Instead of Italy, you're in Holland. She continues the metaphor, allowing for the disappointment of missing out on seeing Italy, like everyone else. But still, she says, once you get acclimated, you might find there is much that is good about Holland.

I think of the stories we tell ourselves, our own personal narratives. They are powerful, and they can be healing. I think of Emily Perl Kingsley, speaking to me across the miles, across the years, through her writing. Here is a woman who does not feel that having a baby with Down syndrome is a great tragedy. Here is a woman offering me a new story, one that is just beginning. For the first time in twenty-four hours, I feel something other than sadness. Emily Perl Kingsley's words spark in me a tiny flicker of hope.

I continue reading. I learn Down syndrome is the most common chromosomal anomaly, occurring once in every 733 births. I learn that during normal cell development, the original cell begins to grow by dividing and duplicating itself over and over. Sometimes, for reasons that are not yet known, the original cell does not divide equally. It continues to grow and duplicate itself, and its error. When the extra genetic material is located at the twenty-first chromosome, it is called trisomy 21, which is also known as Down syndrome, after John Langdon Down, an English physician who first described the condition in 1866.

Although babies with Down syndrome have extra genetic

material at the number 21 chromosome, all of their other chromosomes are normal. In fact, the material in the number 21 chromosome is normal, too—there is just more of it. Which is why babies with Down syndrome are more like typically developing babies than they are different from them. And I learn there is great diversity regarding intelligence, learning styles, physical ability, creativity, and personality, because of the influence of the other forty-six chromosomes in each baby's genetic blueprint.

There are three major types of Down syndrome, and Avery's is the most common, which comprises 95 percent of the diagnoses. It is called nondisjunction trisomy 21, which means chromosome 21 did not disjoin from itself and divide evenly. This happens at the beginning of cell division and the error is copied in each of his cells. There is another form called translocation trisomy 21, where part of the number 21 chromosome breaks off and attaches itself elsewhere, sometimes to the number 14 chromosome, or sometimes to the other number 21 chromosome. The third type of Down syndrome is a rare form called mosaicism, in which the error occurs a bit later in cell division, so only some of the cells contain and perpetuate the trisomy.

The binder has information about support groups, including the National Down Syndrome Society (NDSS). There is a photocopy from their organization called "Myths and Truths." I take it as sort of a pretest, and I fail. I believe all the myths. Down syndrome is not a rare genetic disorder, but a common one. People with Down syndrome are not severely retarded, but fall into the mild-to-moderate range. People with Down syndrome are not always happy (they have a full range of feelings, like everyone else). Down syndrome is not fatal, and 80 percent of adults with Down syndrome live to age 55 or beyond.

The rest of the information in my binder consists of photocopies of newspaper articles with titles like "Special Triumphs" and "A Special Gift" and "Missoula Resident to Be a Bright Light in Times Square." I scan through them, not really reading but getting the idea I have a whole lot more to learn. There are copies of health protocols and growth charts. I notice a help-line phone number for the NDSS. It catches my eye for no other reason than I like the logo. I am too tired to call tonight, but maybe I will later. I pull the page from its plastic sleeve and set it in the binder's front pocket.

The last pages hold color copies of local babies and children with Down syndrome. Each is described by a parent with words full of pride and love, just as any mom or dad would describe any child. I close the book here, my last thoughts not in words but in images, of the faces of beautiful smiling children who also happen to have Down syndrome.

The lights in the house are out, all except my reading lamp. The radio is off. I think of waking Tom, to share this news with him, but decide to let him sleep—there's nothing here that can't wait until morning. I have one thing left to do: I dial the number of the hospital. Jennifer the night nurse answers, and I ask after the babies.

"They're doing great!" she says.

"Okay, thank you," I say. "Good night."

The moon is full and bright across the shimmering water of the lake. I can hear the hum of the refrigerator, I can hear the clicking of the dishwasher as its cycle ends. Everything is in perfect stillness, waiting. Waiting for the babies.

Good night, stars.

Good night, air.

Good night, noises everywhere.


The first thing I notice is that Owen is not here. Our babies are where we left them the day before, but Owen's isolette is gone.

While we were home, something bad came in the night to the crib right next to ours. I know better, but ask anyway.

"Where's the twenty-seven-week baby?" The nurse is the same one as yesterday, the blonde who was eating a bagel and drinking orange juice. Today her bagel has peanut butter on it.

She looks at me, tilts her head, and says, "You know I can't say anything. It's confidential."

And there is more bad news, about Avery. He's been having apnea and bradycardia episodes. The nurse calls them A/B spells. Avery's breathing stops, she tells us; then his heart stops, too.

"So I want to watch his stats. Let him drop to eighty and sixty before I give him any stim. Most docs recommend that—not to stim too early. And I can't let you hold him until we figure this out."

I'm not happy with her plan. It makes me nervous, but like everything else in the NICU, I accept it as the way life has to be.

As if on cue, Avery's stats begin to change. "Here we go," she says almost excitedly.

First it's the respiration monitor, a simple alarm that sounds when more than four seconds pass between inhalations. Without thinking about it, I begin holding my breath, too.

His heartbeat follows, slowing, slowing. These numbers go down in twos, almost gently, the beating of a once strong and mighty force reducing as if it has switched to pumping tar, or is simply running out of batteries. And the pulse-ox monitor begins to sound, its numbers dropping, tumbling down, down.

The nurse reaches for the oxygen tank on her desk, then begins counting. Tom and I stand there, motionless. I'm still holding my breath.

The instant is like the space on a pinhead—finite and yet infinite. I think how Avery's tiny lungs have never held a breath of fresh air. I think how he's never felt the warmth of the summer sun on his cheek. He's never heard the waves crashing on the lakeshore, he's never slept in the crib waiting for him at home.

It's not long enough, I think. His life has not been long

enough. I feel the loss of him already, as if it were inevitable. And I am ashamed of myself, of my hesitance and my fear. I want another chance.

*Breathe, baby, breathe.*

I think of the onesies he has never worn, the hand-knit baby blanket that has never been wrapped around him. I think of Carter, waiting for his life as a big brother to begin. All of it, on hold, until the babies come home. It never occurred to me that one of them might not make it.

I try to slow the beating of my own heart, willing Avery to come back to me. I want another chance to love him better.

I'm having trouble holding my breath. It's been too long. It's not working. I need to do something. I feel helpless, and confused. What should I do? What can I do?

I look at the nurse, who is watching Avery intently. I look at Tom, who is stony and ashen. I look at Avery, small and still as a doll.

*Please, baby, please. Please, come back to me.*

It is Father's Day. There is a child missing, a baby just twenty-seven weeks old gone from the front of the NICU. There is a baby in a purple-and-white knit cap with a haziness about him, suspended somewhere between lungs breathing and heart beating, and not. There is a mother and a father watching it all happen, helpless. A nurse is counting down the seconds, "Ten. Nine. Eight. Seven."

The heart rate is falling: ninety, eighty-eight, eighty-six.

"Six."

The pulse-ox: seventy.

"Five."

Heart rate, eighty. Pulse-ox, sixty.

"Four. Three. Two."

Nearby, there is a baby in a green-and-yellow knit cap who lifts his head and cries, a clear piercing note that breaks the spell—the baby in the purple-and-white cap lifts his head and cries back.

The monitors stop beeping. The stats jump up—heart rate and oxygen saturation levels both return to the nineties; respiration, every two seconds. The nurse puts the tank on her desk. The mother and father stare at each other, dumbfounded, frozen in place like statue people, until finally, the mother remembers to breathe.

# 4

## Home Is Not Where You Thought It Was

When we return from the NICU, I settle Carter in for the afternoon, I speak with Tom awhile, I pump more milk, and then I excuse myself. I get back in the car and drive down the hill to the lake. I park as close as I can. Then I walk slowly, gingerly down the wooded path through gauzy air that smells of smoke from the distant forest fires. Rimmed on the east by the Missions, on the west by low hills rising to Blacktail Peak, and to the north by the Swan and the Whitefish ranges, the water is protected by mountains rising like big-shouldered brothers on every side.

I carefully cross the gravel beach, its cool smooth stones all the colors of the earth—ochre and gray, blue, brown, green, black. I walk until the water reaches my knees; then I kneel down into it. The scar is still fresh across my midsection and the Steri-Strips haven't come off, but I don't care. I fall into the gentle waves, a woman giving herself up. I spread my arms wide, suspended, holding my breath, the difference between floating and drowning merely a matter of inches. For the first time in the day, I begin to shake, not from a chill but from a grief so deep I can't find the tears.

I don't know how to sort out what I'm feeling. Partly, it feels like regret. I wonder why I'd ever wanted more children, and I mourn the loss of our previous life, which now seems unbelievably carefree and lucky. We'd had everything we needed—a house, a beautiful child, each other—why had I wanted more?

There's fear, too, raw and full of adrenaline. Whatever I want or need doesn't matter much in the face of a baby who sometimes doesn't breathe. And Bennett is losing weight. The nurses explained that these setbacks were to be expected; that every baby has to get the kinks worked out before they can be released, but I know differently. The babies need a mother, one who's there with them always, one who can breathe for them and coax milk a drop at a time into their tiny birdlike mouths. The pumping and dripping and beeping machines, the too-sweet smell, the hum of the HVAC, the greenish fluorescent light, the cries, the needles, the blood. The breathing, the not breathing. Each visit starts out fresh and full of hope, and within a few hours I feel dead inside. I stay for as long as I can; then I flee, back to my child and my husband and my lake, leaving the babies behind. They need me, and I'm not there.

I feel sorrow for the loss of Avery as we'd imagined him. It's as if he'd already died, the blond-haired boy who would grow to be six feet tall, strong and strapping, healthy and full of life. It would have been my job to help him grow into a good man—to teach him and his brothers to be strong and masculine like their father, but to be soft, too. Men who knew how to plant a garden, how to bake a loaf of bread, how to hold a baby. We chose for him the name Avery, which means "wise ruler, wise counselor." He would have been a kind, gentle leader: the world would have welcomed such a boy.

And hatred. I hate my weakness. I hate my fear. I hate my selfishness. I hate the NICU, and the cheery nurses in bright colorful caps. I hate the niceties, every "Good morning!" and "You look wonderful!" and the standard response to any question about the babies: "They're doing great!" As if I can't see the state of affairs clearly, as if I'm a child that needs to be handled, or an imbecile.

Which makes me hate the situation most of all—an impossible setup, one that can't be changed or improved, only endured. There are thirteen black *X*s on my calendar. Each time I try to get a release date, I'm told, "Soon, maybe even tomorrow!" by the chipper nurses so that the phrase becomes meaningless, and I stop asking. The doctors are more philosophical: "When they're ready. We know more with each passing day." I ask about having the babies transferred to the hospital in our hometown, which would at least bring them closer to me. But it isn't an option. The local hospital doesn't have the staff or the equipment for round-the-clock neonatal care, which is what the babies require.

Mostly of all, there's hurt. My body is newly split and stitched back together, and I'm bruised. I wonder what I'd done to deserve this trouble, which seems arbitrary and cruel, as if I'd taken a beating for wanting nothing more than what most people want, and yet here I am, returning to the water like some injured animal, circling to home.

Tom is a member of the local volunteer fire department. The VFD holds a garage sale as a fund-raiser each May, and it's the job of the volunteers to set up and run the sale, then dispose of the left-over things afterward. Which is how we came to have a child-size bicycle helmet in the back of the Expedition—it was in a box of unsold garage sale items, destined for the secondhand store. The helmet is round and white and looks like a giant Ping-Pong ball with a strap and a cutout for a face. It's not fashionable, or cool, which is probably why it didn't sell. Carter found it, and without asking either Tom or me, he's begun wearing it. He looks like Ralph from Beverly Cleary's *The Mouse and the Motorcycle*.

I've been making more phone calls. Each conversation gets a little easier. Sometimes, I change it up, to see if I like the results any better. For instance, I try telling people that Avery has trisomy 21. It sounds more technical, medical, and, I think, more knowledge-able. Like we have a handle on things. Plus, trisomy 21 is relatively obscure; there are no preconceived notions about a baby with T21. The news could mean anything. Most people proceed cautiously with, "Is that bad?" To which I answer, "Oh, no, it's nothing at all. Many people have it; you don't realize how common it is until it happens to your baby." Which is true in the literal sense, but saying it this way feels like a lie.

I go back to the regular "Avery has Down syndrome."

There are two versions of the conversation. If the person I call has no knowledge of what's happened—the premature delivery, the NICU—I put the news in the middle of the story. I start by saying, "Well, we had quite a surprise at the beginning of June." Then a quick summary, "My water broke, and despite the doctors' best efforts, the babies couldn't wait. They came early, about seven weeks." I move it right along. "They are still in the hospital, and well, there's one more thing. Avery has Down syndrome." Then I add the final line, "We want them home. They're still in the hospital, and we just want them home." At times I find myself adding the phrase, "If you could, keep a good thought for us."

The second version is for the people who already know the babies are in the NICU. It's a shorter version and goes like this: "We've gotten some tests back on Avery, and we have some unexpected news. He has Down syndrome."

Sometimes people say, "I'm sorry." Sometimes, "Is there anything I can do?" or, "But he's healthy otherwise, right?" Once, "God bless you." None of these reactions bother me. I see in them that no one knows what to say. You can't congratulate us; and yet you don't want to act as if it's the end of the world.

The best reaction is my friend Sarah's. Sarah is my liberal, Ivy League friend. She's tall and blond and statuesque, the type of woman you might be intimidated by until you get to know her and realize she is also thoughtful and sincere. She came to Montana from back east ten years earlier, because she fell in love. Before agreeing to the move, she asked two questions: "Where can I get my hair done?" and "Who's the best ob-gyn?"

Sarah lives with her husband, Ric, and their two young boys

in a remodeled farmhouse on a bench of land that overlooks the lake. Her house sits on two acres that she calls the meadow and that is surrounded by deep purple lilacs.

"I needed to hear your voice," she says over the phone, breathless and apologetic. "I'm sorry for calling. I know you're busy. I just need to know you're okay." We hadn't spoken since I'd gotten home. Telling her, and telling my friend Phyllis, were two of the harder conversations I still needed to have.

"No, no. I've been meaning to call you," I say.

"Now you're scaring me. What's going on?" she says.

"The doctors did some tests on Avery, and we got the results back. He has Down syndrome."

I can hear her begin crying softly, and it makes me cry, too. She's that kind of friend. If you hurt, she hurts. I wanted to spare her but couldn't. She needed to know, and I needed to tell her.

"I love you," she blurts out. We've been friends for seven years and seen each other through sick babies, first babysitters, food allergies, poison ivy, rashes, stomach viruses, birthday parties, and mommies' groups, and yet she's never said that to me before.

"Me, too," I say. "Thanks."

"What can I do?" she says.

"There's one thing," I begin. "Phyllis doesn't know. Can you tell her, and tell her I'll call her in a few days?"

"Sure. Do you want me to tell anyone else? Should I spread the word?" she asks.

"I don't want you to have to do that. It's not your responsibility."

"But people are asking about you. What should I tell them?"

All of a sudden I feel so tired. So very, very tired. "I guess I don't have an answer. I'm sorry. Do whatever you want," I say. "I've got to go."

"Okay, okay. Call if you need anything," she says quietly.

❧

The bills have begun coming to the house. The yellow IV solution costs $6,865. Round-the-clock nursing care, level three, $18,040. There is also a Room-Board charge, $2,079. Each of these expenses are times two, twins. There's my C-section, $6,600. Avery has additional costs: a pathology/cytology report, which I assume was his genetics testing, for $650; and echocardiology, $950, for the examination by a heart specialist, who had called us at home with the greeting, "Good news! You won't be taking an emergency Life Flight to Seattle!"

I read through the statements at night, trying to make sense of them, trying to understand what is happening to our babies and why. It feels odd and a bit invasive, like reading someone else's diary, but I can't help myself. From the insurance company, I learn how much each baby is eating, what supplies they require, everything spelled out down to the last Q-tip. These are things a mother should know without having to look them up, but it's all I have. When I finish with each accounting, I read about Avery.


I Google "Down syndrome": there are 2,370,000 entries. I scan sites. Many are Web pages for parents' groups across the country, even the world—there are Down syndrome groups in Mexico, Ireland, Germany, even one in New South Wales. Soon enough, I realize the pages are mostly similar. They refer parents to NDSS and NADS; usually there is a copy of or link to Emily Perl Kingsley's essay "Welcome to Holland"; often there are family photos, which I examine closely, trying to find a child who might look like Avery.

I notice unimportant and random things, too: that the site for the Down Syndrome Association of Los Angeles has a special section for casting agents; that there are organizations with unusual names, such as Einstein Syndrome, or Up Syndrome, or Uno Mas!, which remind me of the short time I was telling people Avery had trisomy 21. It seems that other parents have trouble finding the right words, too. One site has the same information as the others, plus it's won two dozen awards—the Riverbend Down Syndrome Parent Support Group. It's too much to take in all at once, so I bookmark it.

I learn that the current, preferred terminology is Down syndrome. If you see the condition referred to as Down's, or Down's Syndrome, or Down Syndrome, you are probably dealing with outdated information. The current thinking is that a child is a child first, so instead of a "Down's baby," you would say "a baby with Down syndrome." The second phrase is much longer and a bit awkward, but I understand the desire to find language that honors the spirit of the child, and that also includes the medical diagnosis, whatever that might be.

I also learn that there is no 's in Down syndrome, as it is a genetic condition named after the man who first described it; it doesn't belong to him, so it is not a possessive form. And "syndrome" is not capitalized, as it is not a proper noun.

Finally, sometimes Down syndrome is abbreviated as DS, which is helpful but a bit confusing, as DS can also be an abbreviation in cyberspace for Dear Son, which in my case is accurate, since Avery is a DS and has DS, too. Until I figured this out, I thought I'd hit upon one hotbed after another of families living with Down syndrome.

Many of the sites have a reference section, and I take note of the books that come up again and again. One of them is the familiar *Babies with Down Syndrome*, which is hidden in our bookshelf. There's also *A Parent's Guide to Down Syndrome: Toward a Brighter Future*, by Siegfried M. Pueschel, and *Understanding Down Syndrome: An Introduction for Parents*, by Cliff Cunningham. I order the two we don't have, pay with a credit card, click off the computer, and go to bed.

❧

"You know campers, Mommy?" Carter asks. "People live in them and travel all over the world." He has on his secondhand helmet, and he's strapped in his car seat in the middle of the big back row. Don and Joyce have gone home to catch up with their lives; the baby carriers are in the garage, because it's too depressing driving around with empty car seats. We're on our way to the hospital, and Tom just passed a pickup truck pulling a travel trailer.

"Sure, honey, people do that. Would you like to do that?" I say.

"No," Carter says. "I love our *home*." When he says "home," he draws the word out dramatically for emphasis.

We drive down the highway, the three of us, still a family but slightly off-kilter now, a bit broken. Neither Tom nor I have asked Carter about the helmet, and I don't think we will. I understand it intuitively, and I think it's the most honest reaction to the last few weeks that anyone has had. I wish I could wear a helmet around, too, and maybe some big hockey pads.

We drive along the base of the mountains through the fertile green valley. Black cows graze the hillsides, their gangly-legged calves racing between and beneath them. We pass the little county roads that shoot off from the main highway, as familiar to me now as the lines on the palm of my hand—Beaverhead Road, Duck Road, Kicking Horse Road. Eagle Pass Road, Gunlock Road, Post Creek Road. The green highway sign that reads, MISSOULA—40 MI. An old Ford flatbed passes us on the left, loaded with a round bale, and bits of grass hay flake off into the air like green rain.

More driving, past the National Bison Range and the turnoff to Moiese. The willows along the creek beds and the drainages are blooming bright yellow. I see a cluster of far-off brown dots the size of little chocolate chips, bison or cows moving in the distance. We pass barbed-wire fence, abandoned buildings, old homesteads. I'm in a reflective mood. I think about hard times, and trouble. A baby like Avery, born a hundred years ago, would have had a very different life. But then, if we lived a hundred years ago, I wouldn't be thinking about any of this. I'd be one of the statistics—women lost to childbirth. I'd be dead.

My eyes wander to the right and I see, improbably, a windmill. Like the black-and-white-and-gray photocopy in my binder, like the little houses you might see in Holland. There it sits, right next to the railroad tracks. I swivel my head as we pass, staring. It must have always been there, unseen by me. But I'm not sure. Everything has become suspect lately.

"What is it?" Tom asks.

I can't explain, and I'm not convinced I really saw it, so I say, "Nothing. It's nothing."

When we reach the hospital parking lot, Tom pulls up to the entrance and drops me off. He and Carter are going to a nearby park to play with the new Wiffle ball and bat. I head inside and make my usual stops—first to the bathroom, then to the front desk, where I'm buzzed in, then to the washing station, finally to the Breastfeeding Room. All this, even before I see them.

I hold my babies, I rock them, I kiss them. When they are in my arms, we are as we were meant to be—three pieces of a puzzle fit back together. I forget the trouble, and for a while, everything is all right. This well-being is temporary and fleeting. It doesn't last; I begin to feel trapped. Already, I miss Tom and Carter. I pass the babies back to the nurse, Carol.

Each has a clipboard with a paper on which information for the day is recorded. The chart looks like a long rectangular sheet of graph paper crammed full of pluses, dashes, backslashes, and numbers. There's also a place for comments, which are written in medical jargon and abbreviations. I ask to see the charts. Sometimes I can; sometimes I can't. I always ask, anyway.

"Sure," she says. "Why not?"

I notice that the babies have been getting more breast milk, and that today there wasn't enough. Avery was given formula. I blink hard a few times, swallow, and continue scanning through the numbers. I see a spot on the bottom that I'd never noticed before. It reads, *M/contact.* Next to it there is a series of dashes—negatives. Then for the four half hours I've been in the hospital, there are pluses. I turn the pages back to the previous day. A sea of minuses. The day before that. More minuses. The nurses have been keeping track of everything, including me. Minuses everywhere. No, no, no, no. Not enough milk. No mother.

I put the chart down and push toward the exit, where I peel off the hospital gown that covers my street clothes and toss it toward the laundry bin. I wave my hand in the air at the camera watching the locked door, and it opens. I rush down the long wide corridor. My heart is beating fast and my eyes are watering. I make one stop at the vending machine, plunking in three quarters and a dime, to buy Carter's cookies, the pink-and-white-frosted animal crackers that he calls sparkle cookies after the sprinkles on top. I promised him I would get some, and I do. Then I am out, into the sun.

There is no air as fresh as the first breath outside the NICU. I'm like a whale after a deep dive, surfacing in a great, arcing blast. I gulp it in, let it fill me up, let it push out the NICU. I hear the engine of a bus arriving at the hospital entrance, the *whoosh* of the brakes, the squeak of the door. I smell the asphalt heating in the summer sun, and engine exhaust tinged with gasoline. I see bright pink flowers in the beds bordering the grass, and an airplane flying low in the sky. These sensations are nothing, and they are everything—they are the stuff of life, the real world, a world my babies have not yet seen.

The only place to wait for Tom and Carter is a bench at the bus stop, and I sit, as if I were nobody, as if I were just another woman looking for a ride.


An oversize wooden basket sits on the porch next to the gas grill, waiting for us when we arrive home. In it is a box full of preemie clothes, and a note from Sarah. It reads: "Baby stuff—infant car seat, BabyBjörn, bouncy chair, baby swing, Gymini (baby gym), coming soon . . . high chair! Also Kelty pack. These are yours, if you want them. Thinking of you. Call when you can. Love, Sarah." Inside the house, the red light on the answering machine is blinking—a message from Phyllis. She says that she's spoken with Sarah, and that she's praying for us.

I've know Phyllis as long as I've known Sarah. When I think of Phyllis, I think of a story about a symbol drawn by hobos on fence posts and doorways—a cat with a giant heart inside, which lets everyone know the lady of the house is a kindhearted woman, likely to provide a meal or a warm place to sleep. Phyllis gathers children in need of a boost and teaches them to make music. She finds homes for stray pianos, often with families who can't even pay her for the lessons. It's impossible to give her anything, because she'll turn around and give it to someone else "who needs it more than me." She bakes marvelous loaves of braided bread, two at a time—one to keep, and one to share. Phyllis is a kindhearted woman.

I dial her number.

"Hello! It's me," I say. "Is this a good time?"

"Well, duh," she says, "of course it is. It's so good to hear your voice."

"Yeah. It's good to hear yours, too," I say.

"How are you?" she asks.

"Okay. I'm trying not to think too much. I want to get the babies home. We can figure out the rest of it then."

"What do you need?" she asks.

"Well, I have a silly question. I can't seem to get my milk up. Is there anything I should try?"

"I've heard there's an herbal tea you can drink. I can't remember what it's called, something like Mother's Milk Tea. And I also heard you can drink nonalcoholic beer for the hops—that's supposed to help. But the main thing is rest and relaxation. I don't know how to help you with that. I bet you're running yourself ragged," she says.

"No. I thought it would be so busy with two babies, and so happy. Mostly, it's waiting. I feel like I have empty arms. But what can you do?" I say.

"Eat chocolate. That, or get a new haircut. You know what I always say, 'If you can't change your life, change your hair.' Chocolate is cheaper."

"I'm still huge. People think I haven't had the babies yet. And none of my clothes fit. The maternity stuff is like wearing a circus tent without the pole, and I don't know if I'll ever fit in my normal clothes again," I say.

"Let me get you some things to borrow. I have two of every size and color in the rainbow. I'll get a box to Sarah and she can bring it out to your house."

"That would be terrific. I keep wearing the same two outfits: I have a pair of black pants that fit if I turn over the waistband, and I have a dress that cinches in. The nurses switch shifts every two days so I'm hoping no one's noticed."

"Can I do anything else?" she asks.

"Keep a good thought," I say.

"I've already added you to the prayer chain. Our whole church is praying for you."

"I don't know what to say."

"Don't say anything. You'd do the same for me," she says.

I have one more phone call I need to make, to our neighbor Cathy. She's pregnant with her second child. I call, but no one answers. I leave a message on the machine, saying we are home, the babies are still in Missoula, and I have more news, too, if Cathy can call me back.


As the days pass, the lake warms and the summer houses fill. To the right of the public beach, a white-haired man lives with his elderly wife. Sometimes their adult children visit, bringing almost-grown children of their own. To the left, there is a rickety little blue house, its yard filled with too many cars, overflowing trash cans, and a permanently parked fifth-wheel RV for extra guests.

I'm in the middle of the two places, floating in the water off the public beach, watching three teenage boys clambering in and out of the back of a speedboat. Blond, tanned, and strong, close enough in age and appearance to be brothers. They are beautiful, full of summer and youth and themselves. Sadness washes over me. They are three. They are my boys, the family I imagined, the family that is not mine.

The boys are playing and roughhousing as the speedboat drifts in the shallows. One of them falls into the driver's seat, steadies himself, and grabs the wheel. *Oh, no,* I think. *Oh, no. You're not old enough to drive a speedboat.* And then there are the other two, swimming in back near the motor, near the propeller that will begin to spin and slice if the boy turns the ignition.

My mouth is filled with the sharp metallic taste of fear.

*This is how it happens,* I think. This is how bad things happen. Everything is fine one moment, and the next, it's broken, hopelessly broken. I want to shout out a warning, but I know better. I am just some strange woman made crazy by her own grief.

I turn my back to them, and haul myself up and out of the water. I can hear the engine catch, then roar away. There are no screams, there's no blood. I turn again and see the wake of the boat, an upside-down V that points to the boys standing in the bow three across, laughing and whooping, their shoulders golden in the sun.

A woman makes her way over to me from the rickety blue house. She is about my age, but tan and slim. I assume she is the mother of the boys.

"You're not supposed to drive down here," she says. No introduction, no hello. "There's a sign now. No cars." She points to a white board with stick-on letters attached to a metal pole in their yard. "You didn't see that?" she says.

I hadn't.

"No. I didn't notice it," I say. "I'm sorry."

"You have to leave. You can't drive down here anymore." She points to my car, waggling her finger at it as if it were completely out of order to park a car in a parking spot.

Any previous summer, I might have behaved differently. I might have asked her who she was, and how she came to be involved. I might have asked who gave her the authority to set new rules and enforce them. I might have been forthright, or I might have tried to befriend her, to find some common ground.

But not today.

Today, it makes perfect sense. Of course the rules are changed. Everything is changed.

I look at her. Three sons.

*You silly woman*, I think.

*You silly, stupid woman.*

*You have everything, and you don't even see it. You don't appreciate it. Until it's gone, and then it's too late.*

*You can never get it back.*

*It's all your fault.*

I say nothing. Of course I should leave. I deserve this. This is my new life. Nothing good will ever come again.

*You stupid woman.*

*Go.*

I leave, and don't come back.


When I arrive at the NICU the next day, the babies are gone. They're not in their isolettes by the front window; they're not in the back, by the refrigerator. I panic. I spin around and begin my search for them again, this time in earnest. I ignore the NICU protocol and begin looking right at babies, peering in isolettes, reading name tags.

A nurse takes my arm and asks, "Can I help you?"

"Where are my babies?" I ask. "Where are the Groneberg twins?"

"Let me check. Sit here and wait. I'll be right back." She pulls out a swivel chair and deposits me in it, then disappears.

I wait. I feel responsible, as if I've somehow caused this. I broke the chain that kept us all together, all intact. I never called Cathy, just left a message. I was cross with Carter at breakfast. I'd been taking everything for granted again. I'd had so much, and still, I didn't see it. Stupid, stupid.

The nurse returns.

"The babies have been moved up to Peds. That's on the third floor. Get your things, and your milk from the fridge, and I'll show you," she says.

"Are they okay?" I ask.

"They're doing great!"

I collect myself and follow the nurse out through the locked door, back down the wide corridor to the elevator near the gift shop. She presses 3. As we wait, we're joined by a woman in jeans and a tank top holding a bouquet of balloons in children's colors—blue, red, yellow—tied with curling ribbons. We ride together to the third floor.

At the front desk, the nurse introduces me. "She's the mother of the twins," she tells the woman behind the front desk, then turns to me and says, "I'll leave you here. They'll take care of you."

The woman with the balloons walks past the front desk and down the hall. She already knows where she is going. I don't. I stand there, shifting my weight from one foot to the other, my little blue insulated cooler filled with milk, my plastic bag of attachments for the hospital's breast pump. Everything is changing again and I'm trying not to think bad thoughts.

There are no locked doors up here. It's quieter. There are windows in every room. I can see the sky, which is the washed-out blue of faded denim. The nurses are not wearing scrubs, like in the NICU, but street clothes and colorful lab coats with swirling patterns of cartoon puppies and kittens playing tug-of-war and the words *Happy Woof Day*. A fish tank bubbles in the corner, and the walls are painted with a bright, jungle-themed mural. Tigers and lions and giraffes and a zebra. I try to think of reasons why we might have been moved; nothing sinister comes to mind. It feels like we've gotten a promotion.

A nurse finishes typing at a keyboard and walks out from behind the front desk. She's young and has a bounce to her step when she walks, which makes her ponytail swing back and forth. I follow her down the hall and into a room on the right, where I can see my babies, dressed in little outfits I don't recognize, sleeping together in what looks like a clear plastic tub.

The fish-finder machines are here, but the isolettes are gone. The IVs are gone, and there are no bags of yellow solution *drip drip drip*-ing. The stomach tubes are gone, and for the first time, I can see their little faces clearly. I feel like I might burst with happiness. I want to hug everyone.

"They look like real babies now, don't they?" says the ponytail nurse, interpreting my thoughts.

"Yes," I say. "When did this happen?"

"The doc said they could be transferred up here this morning. We just got them settled," she says, and adds, "This is your new nurse. She'll help you."

"It's all good, isn't it?" I ask of the second nurse, afraid to believe it. "I mean, it seems like a step up?"

"You could look at it like that, yes," she says. She's a plain woman, with mousy brown hair pulled back into a bun. She's wearing the royal blue scrubs of the NICU, and has big oval glasses.

"I put them together so they can have their twin time," she says. "They need to be together. This baby"—she points to Bennett—"this baby will lead the way. This one"—she points to Avery—"will follow. You're lucky you have two of them." She doesn't speak to me as if I were a child; rather, she speaks to me as if I might be able to handle whatever she's got to say.

"Does this mean they will be going home soon?" I ask, thinking this time I might get a real answer.

"Yes. We're going to get you out of here," she says.

"How will it happen?" I ask. It feels a bit ridiculous, like we're conspirators hatching a plan, and she's filling me in on the details.

"First," she says, "they have to be able to maintain their body temperatures. That's why they're out of the isolettes. Next," she continues, "they have to be able to hold their weights. Can I ask you something?"

"Sure, what?"

"You signed a form that said you wanted to breast-feed. If you change to bottle feed, they'll go home faster. Did you know that?"

I didn't. But it made sense. The only practice the babies get at eating is when I'm here; all the rest of the feedings are by tube or syringe. If I change to bottles, the nursing staff can feed them even when I'm not here.

"Let's do it," I say.

"Another thing," she says. "Avery is still having A/B spells. If you and your husband learn infant CPR, he could go home with a portable monitor and supplemental oxygen. Did you know that?"

"No," I say. "Tom already knows CPR. He's with the volunteer fire department. Is that it?"

"You'll have to room in with them overnight so you can learn their care routines. You might think about making arrangements for that. And the babies will have to pass a car seat test. We put them in their carriers and monitor them, to make sure they can handle the drive home. You should bring yours in and have them ready," she says.

"I will," I say. "Thank you for telling me all this."

"Somebody should," she says. "Might as well be me. I know what it's like," she adds. "I had a daughter with CP. No one would tell me anything. I had to figure it out on my own. That's why I went into nursing."

"How old is your daughter?" I ask.

"She died five years ago."

"I'm sorry," I say.

"It's okay. You get a thick skin," she says. "You'll get one, too. You'll see."

I don't want a thick skin. I want my babies home, and anything beyond that seems like too much to think about. I can't wait to tell Tom. We'll have to call Don and Joyce and ask them to come back; more phone calls to share the good news; we'll have to get the house ready, and the shopping done.

After all the worrying, all the doubt, after all the sadness, and the waiting, we are finally going home. At last, there is so much to do.

# 5

❧

# Caffeine

It's three o'clock in the afternoon and Tom and I are discussing the merits of caffeine. The coffeemaker is dripping out a fresh pot, and as it spits and sputters, the kitchen is filled with the steamy aroma of Folgers or Maxwell House or whatever brand is on sale. Since the babies have come home, Tom and I have turned into caffeine addicts. If I had time to dream, it would be about shiny espresso machines and tiny cups of liquid the color and thickness of tar. Avery joins us in our habit. He was released from the NICU with a portable monitor, just as our last nurse had predicted, and also with a prescription for pediatric caffeine called Cafcit to "perk him up." We have to search all over northwest Montana to keep his dose (.45 ml by mouth twice a day) in supply. Each pharmacist I call is surprised by my request, asking, "Now why in the world would you need *that*?"

When I'd think about the babies coming home, it was always both of them together. It didn't happen that way. When Dr. Rosquist told me Bennett would be first, I thought I'd heard her wrong. Bennett, the baby who'd had trouble eating, trouble sleeping, trouble growing, was ready to be released before Avery.

"You mean Avery, right?"

"No. Bennett."

"He's ready?" I didn't want to press my luck, but I couldn't believe it.

"Yes. You'll need to stay overnight, we'll do the car seat test, and then you're set," she said.

"But what about Avery?" I asked.

"He still needs to stay."

My mind began racing. I hadn't ever considered the possibility that one baby would stay and one would come home. It seemed very wrong. While they'd both been in the NICU, my main consolation was knowing they had each other. Now that wouldn't be the case. I tried to think of options.

"Could we bring Avery to the hospital near our home? Would they take just one?"

Dr. Rosquist shook her head, no.

"Could Bennett stay until Avery was stronger?"

Again she shook her head, no.

I was grasping for a way to make sense of this news. I wanted to feel happy. We'd at least have one baby home. But I felt as if we were abandoning Avery, leaving our weakest child to fend for himself. My eyes filled with tears.

"I hadn't planned on this. I really wanted them to be together. Could I room in with Bennett?"

Again, she shook her head. "Once he's released, we can't let him back into the NICU."

"But he's not really in the NICU. We're in Peds," I bargained. "Wouldn't that be okay?"

Again, no. "Technically, he's in the NICU. Sometimes parents stay in a motel nearby," she offered.

"Who would watch Bennett while I was here?" I said, thinking aloud.

"Maybe a friend?" She shrugged, and I could tell that these matters were my problems, not hers. I wanted to point out that siblings of children in the PICU were in and out of the rooms all day. How was Bennett any different? But it felt as if I'd reached the end of the conversation with her. I couldn't help but think, *If you were a mother, you'd know how ridiculous this is.* There were no good options.

I called Tom. "Well, it's good news and it's bad news," I began. "What do you want first?"

"Good news."

"Bennett's getting released tomorrow," I said.

"What's the bad news?"

"Avery's staying." As I spoke, my voice cracked. Tom noticed.

"Jen, it's okay. It'll be okay. I thought you were going to tell me something *really* bad."

"But how can we do this? It's impossible. They won't let me stay with Bennett. They won't let Bennett stay until Avery's ready. They won't let Avery go to St. Joseph's. . . . It's a mess. I don't know how we can manage it."

"It'll be okay. I'll call my folks. You bring Bennett home and I'll go down for Avery every day."

I hadn't thought of that. "Really?" I asked. "You'd do that?"

"Of course."

"Wow. Okay, then." I felt almost giddy. Now we had a plan. "I'll get done here and be home soon. Tomorrow I need to stay overnight, and then hopefully Bennett will come home with me."

For a while after we were married, before we had children, Tom and I lived on the wide, open grasslands of eastern Montana. The air was dry and smelled of sage, even in the winter. One night found us at the home of the minister of the Methodist church, where we'd been invited for dinner. We suspected a recruitment effort might take place.

The minister was a curly-haired, gray-bearded man in his

midfifties. In addition to God, he loved carpentry, organic farming, and small animal husbandry. He asked that we call him Bob. He and his wife had two children, a boy and a girl, both grown. We ate a meal of lasagna and a salad made from garden lettuce, and not once did he speak about his church. When the dishes had been cleared and stacked, he asked us to follow him down to the basement, where he kept his wine-making supplies.

He led us through a half-size door next to the refrigerator, down steep steps, into a great black cavern. Bob pulled a chain and a single lightbulb illuminated the basement, a great, deep space that was shored up with timbers and metal pipes.

"We dug this ourselves," he said proudly, stretching his arms out and pointing at the four corners. "We wanted a basement but couldn't afford the heavy equipment. So we did it ourselves, one bucket at a time."

"That's incredible," Tom said. "How long did it take you?"

"About three years. But look what it got us." Again, he swung his arms through the space. One bucket at a time. I couldn't imagine it. I'm not a person of great patience. And faith—how would you know you weren't going to collapse your house? I was thinking all these things, wondering how a person could manage it, when I realized that perhaps this basement was his preaching. Maybe this was his way of telling us about himself and his church, about foundations and faith.

"It's amazing" was all I could say.

I'm thinking about Bob the minister's basement as I watch Bennett sleep in his car seat. When I returned to the hospital I brought his going-home outfit, his baby carrier, and six cloth diapers. I also packed a bag for me, and the breast pump, and the little plastic bags for the milk, and the stickers for the bags, but only for Avery, since Bennett wouldn't be here after today. I hadn't slept yet, because of nerves and worry and sadness over leaving Avery behind, and also because of the hospital sounds—an announcement that the Life Flight would be landing for something called a Code Blue; carts wheeling up and down the hallway; the beeping of monitors; the hum and click of the HVAC. And there was something else, which may or may not have been real. All night long, beneath the other night noises, like an echo without the initial "Hello," I thought I heard the faintest sound of children crying.

Avery is in the room with us, but soon we would be leaving. Bennett is strapped into the car seat, no longer in his green-and-yellow knit cap, which belongs to the hospital, but in a white one of ours with a teddy bear on it. Wires connecting him to his monitors come through the front of his outfit, the exact one I'd brought Carter home in four years ago—a little white footed sleeper, with cuffs that fold over the sleeves to make mittens. On Carter, who was eight pounds, ten ounces, the sleeper had been tight. On Bennett, who is barely five pounds, it looks huge.

Even the car seat was too big; the nurse, a new one, young and earnest, showed me how to roll the cloth diapers into logs to place alongside Bennett, to position his head, his body, his legs so they were snug. In this hospital, all babies have to be able to maintain themselves in their car seat for the length of time it will take for them to reach home, which for us is an hour and a half.

As I sit and wait, my eyes are glued to the monitors. The car seat test is the last thing Bennett has to pass to be released, and it's the longest ninety minutes of my life. Each time Bennett moves, the pulse-ox goes off, and I think, *This is it. They'll tell me we have to stay.* And then I think, *Well, fine, then Avery won't be alone.* I've never wanted something, and not wanted something so much at the same time. Which is why I'm thinking about Bob the minister's basement.

One bucket at a time.

The morning continues to pass, the minutes slowly adding up, until we are done. But the nurse is nowhere to be found. I consider leaving. I could unhook Bennett, gather our belongings, and walk out the revolving front door into the hazy summer heat. My heart sinks. Avery. I consider unhooking him, too. We will go. I will take them. Is this how it happens? Is this how a mother ends up on the nightly news, in a high-speed car chase, for stealing her babies? But where would I go? I would only go home. And I would drive carefully, and slowly. I am a chicken.

So I wait.

Eventually the nurse reappears with papers to sign, and forms to take home, and a certificate saying Bennett has passed his hearing test. She hands me a mauve plastic bin filled with baby-care items: little packets of ointment and gauze and tiny syringes; a plastic baby brush, a paper tape measure, three tiny diapers. It's the flotsam and jetsam of Bennett's early life, none of it amounting to much. There aren't any vases of flowers to pack up, no stuffed animals or heart-shaped boxes of chocolates or baby cards. I do not leave the hospital in a wheelchair with Mylar balloons trailing behind me, as I did with Carter. This time, I walk out alone, the overnight bag and the little plastic bin in my left arm, the car seat holding Bennett in my right. What is significant here is not what I carry, but what I leave behind: a little red-faced baby in a purple-and-white cap who sometimes forgets to breathe.

Twelve days after Bennett was released, Tom brought Avery home. He packed an overnight bag for himself and chose a going-home outfit for Avery. He took bags of milk for Avery in my little blue cooler, as he had most days for the nearly two weeks he was Avery's primary caregiver. He took a refresher infant CPR class, and he learned how to use the supplemental oxygen, and the little black monitor for Avery's A/B spells, all with the understanding that he would teach me, which he did.

He did all of these things and more: he began washing the dishes and cleaning up the kitchen every night; he sorted out the bottles each morning and evening, telling me how many to make for each baby; he began reading to Carter at bedtime; he washed and folded laundry. He did this work without my asking, and without complaint. In fact, he seemed to be handling our new life better than me. His way with Avery was accepting and forgiving. Where I found fault in Avery's raggedy breathing, or saw weakness in his sputtering heartbeat, Tom didn't. What Avery gave was gentleness, and Tom returned it.

On the day of Avery's release, we got more bad news. He failed the hearing test in his left ear. But when Tom walked in the door holding Avery in his car seat, the black portable monitor with its red blinking light slung over his shoulder, both of them smelling of sour milk from Avery's spit-up on the ride home, the hearing test seemed like a very small blow, almost inconsequential compared to the fact that we were all, finally, home.

Smoke from the forest fires is thick and white and rolls in from the north across the lake. It's a bad fire year and there are two burning near us—the Robert Fire, and the Apgar Mountain fire. Though it's hot, we keep the windows closed against the smoke. There are white cotton diapers everywhere, used for burp cloths or rolled up to keep the babies safe in their seats. In the refrigerator, there's an entire shelf devoted to milk: four Avent bottles for Bennett, because the nipple is the only one he can manage, four preemie bottles from the hospital for Avery, because these are the ones he prefers, and four sippies of chocolate milk for Carter, so he can feel included. Each of the babies' bottles holds three ounces of mostly breast milk, sometimes Enfamil with Lipids. We go through eight bottles in twelve hours, or sixteen in a day. Each one emptied feels like an accomplishment—we are growing, one bottle at a time.

Tom's parents have come back to help us. Don makes runs across the state for Avery's Cafcit, which costs $300 for a week's supply, an expense that's not covered by our insurance. Another cost that we are covering is Avery's monitor, $358 each week. I'd be more concerned about these out-of-pocket expenses if they had come first—but I'd become numb to the many thousands of dollars that the NICU cost, so that anything less seems like a good deal.

The baby books advise me to keep track of diapers, which is so impossible it's funny. I can't even remember what day it is. I move from one thing to the next, one task in front of me to another, and in this way we are surviving. I pump at three, six, nine, and twelve. I only remember this because it's multiples of three and I have three children. I sleep in snatches, whenever I can. My head is constantly throbbing and I pop ibuprofen or acetaminophen like Tic Tacs.

There is Tom, and Carter, there are the babies. Home life and chores. I'm splitting myself four ways, more ways. It's a fractured life, all this multitasking. I feel like a Picasso.

Grandpa takes long meanders with Carter, or builds complicated cities on the LEGO table. Grandma is the only one who can get Bennett to take a bottle. Otherwise, he has decided that he prefers to breast-feed. Avery is the opposite. He squirms and wriggles when I try to get him to latch on, and looks up at me with confusion, as if saying, *Now what in the world am I supposed to do with this?* It feels like another setback, another thing to overcome.

I take *Babies with Down Syndrome: A New Parents' Guide* from the bookshelf, promising myself that I'll only look at the chapter about daily baby care. I turn to the section called "Breast or Bottle Feeding," and begin reading. The first sentence assures the reader that babies like Avery can breast-feed, but as I continue, I see words like "physical characteristics might affect how they eat" and "difficulty" and "weaker suck." I feel discouraged, so I go to the bookshelf and pull out *The Womanly Art of Breastfeeding*, which I'd used with Carter. Babies with Down syndrome are mentioned in a chapter called "Problems at the Beginning." I see phrases like "loving home environment" and "the baby with Down syndrome responds readily." But I also read, "poor sucking reflex" and "extra help and patience." I hesitate. It seems like a lot of work, and I'm not sure I'm up to it. I have misgivings. In the end, maybe he won't be able to do it.

I justify my doubt by telling myself that Avery has a clear preference for the bottle. He's the one who rejected me, not the other way around. But I'm secretly relieved. I don't know what to do with a baby like Avery. Around him, I feel anxious and unsure and inadequate, and I don't like these feelings.

On the refrigerator is a calendar that has phone numbers scribbled across the top and in the margins. There are black $X$s through the days that are done, and stapled to the pages are charts of the babies' feedings: 2:30 a.m. both, 5:30 B, 6:15 A, 8:00 B, 8:30 A, 9:00 B, 10:00 A, 11:00 B, 11:30 A.

Avery's monitor looks like a classic black Coach purse, only inside is a box that reads and records his heart rate—its wires and electrodes are attached to his chest with tape that gives him a blistery red rash. When it's working, a green light blinks soundlessly. When it can't get a reading, or if you accidentally disconnect it while changing a diaper, the noise resembles a fire alarm going off. So far, we have had no actual alarms, only false ones.

Tom has begun sleeping in the living room on the couch, with Avery in a portable Pack 'n Play crib beside him, and the supplemental oxygen tanks and their clear plastic tubing stacked in the corner. When the monitor goes off, he can reset it without waking Carter or Bennett. He's the expert on all things Avery.

When I hold Avery, I inspect him. I hate that I do this to him; I don't do it with Bennett. But I can't seem to help myself. I look deep into his eyes, which are darker blue than his brothers'. His nose turns up at the end, a little button nose. His ears are smaller.

His skin is unusual too, almost papery. His neck is thicker, and not as strong as Bennett's. He's floppier.

Sometimes I want that neck to be different. We could work on it. Find a way to change it. Make it stronger. Make it better. Or we could hide it. Bundle it up, wear turtlenecks. Sometimes I want to wake up and have it all gone, like a bad dream, like I tell Carter—*Wake up, honey. It's okay now. It's all better.*

I'm so incredibly tired. It's noon and I feel as if I've got cement blocks for arms and legs. If I stop moving, I'll fall asleep. I caught myself dozing off while sitting with Bennett. Avery is asleep; he should be good for two hours. I put Bennett in the swing, which might buy me an hour. There's only Carter. Please, please, please, come lie down with Mommy. I lock the doors, pile all the couch cushions and bed pillows on the family room rug. I close the drapes. Everything is quiet. Carter leans into me, spooning. I'm drifting off . . . Avery's awake.

I go to him, hold him. My feelings for him are so complicated. I touch him less, because he's not breast-feeding. I change him less; usually that goes to whoever is feeding him. He's Tom's baby, really. I barely know him. He's so soft, softer than other babies. His chin quivers when he cries. I want to love him, I do. I don't know what's wrong with me. I have the heart of a stone.

Phyllis dropped off a box of clothes with Sarah, who drove it out to our house, kind of a Pony Express of fashion. Phyllis loves bargains. She also has four sisters, with whom she shares clothes. I've never seen her wear the same thing twice.

In her box for me, as promised, are a dozen different outfits in many sizes and colors. I try them on throughout the day, around the feedings and between diaper changes, in a one-woman show: a ruffled pink blouse that makes my breasts look huge; a geometric black-and-red print dress that reminds me of my mother, who loves to wear red; a pair of purple leggings and a purple-and-teal top that makes me feel like Olivia Newton-John in her "Let's Get Physical" phase.

Each new getup is a surprise, like taking a little vacation from myself, trying on all these new possibilities: Who might I be if I wore long gauzy dresses? What about the woman wearing bright bold colors? Or the mysterious woman, dressed all in black? What if I wore nothing but green?

When I'd learned I was pregnant with twins, for the first time in my life I painted my toenails bright red. I was feeling bold and brave, wildly happy. Red seemed right: the color of a bouncy ball, the color of a balloon, the color of a pie cherry hanging in the sunlight. I was so round and ripe I couldn't see past my belly, and Tom had to help me finish the pinky toes.

But when the babies came too soon, I began to hate my red toes, my brashness. The red of my toes reminded me of the color of blood. It was a bull's-eye for disaster. I kept my feet covered in socks until I was able to remove the red with a cotton ball and chemicals that smelled to me like the NICU. I became a woman of no polish. Sensible. Silent. Easy to overlook.

I still feel the need to vanish, all these weeks later. So despite my daylong fashion show, the clothes I choose from Phyllis's box are more of the same. A cream-colored tunic with a satin ribbon around the neck and a thermal-knit top with a tiny pattern of pale blue morning glories. Black stretch pants and a pair of Capri-length jeans. A navy blue–and-white-striped long-sleeved shirt. An oversize white oxford and a short-sleeved denim shirt. Quiet, unassuming clothes for a quiet, unassuming woman; someone I hope will pass by unnoticed.


Avery's on his third outfit. Bennett won't quit crying. Carter is squirrelly and keeps asking me for candy. There are too many children here and not enough grown-ups.

What was I thinking?

We could have gone to Italy. We could have taken a tour of the vineyards, and sat in a piazza sipping Pellegrino with lime. It would have been our own little *Under the Tuscan Sun*, but we'd have added a lovely towheaded, potty-trained little boy.

That, or we could have gotten a new living room set. A soft leather couch the color of milk chocolate, and an oversize chair with a matching ottoman to replace the faded, stained ten-year-old green couch that has a rip in the left cushion, and the mismatched ottoman with stuffing splitting out of the corner.

Instead, I wanted a baby.

I've never worked so hard just to be behind. I'm constantly falling short.

Tom's folks have returned to their home, as they must. Tom is gone on a brief publicity tour for his book. It's the children and me, for the first time, on our own. I knew this day would come, inevitably. I hadn't expected it to be so hard.

The piles of laundry, the stacks of dishes, the shopping, the feedings, the changings are never-ending. I need a maid, a wet nurse, a nanny, a tutor. I need a personal shopper, an assistant, a chef, a trainer. A massage therapist, a manicurist, a hairdresser.

And I need them all yesterday.

I watch television constantly, day and night, just to hear the sound of adult voices. I'm addicted to the Tour de France. The cyclists have support vans that roll up beside them when they are injured, or winded, or have broken a spoke. I need a support van. A mother's support van following alongside me wherever I go, full of helpful people popping out whenever they are needed. Want a nap? Here we are. Need to use the toilet? Take your time. Shower? No problem. How about a paper cup of Gatorade and a splash of cool water in the face?

Instead, there's just me, one woman who smells of spit-up and sweat, breast milk and baby poop; a neglected four-year-old;

and two wailing babies. I don't think they even know why they are crying—only that one is, so the other one cries, too.

This ship is sinking fast.

I have: three hundred Huggies Supremes in the tiny packs, dozens of them, given to us as baby gifts by the volunteer fire department. A freezer full of meals made in disposable tin pans wrapped in foil, the contents written in black Sharpie, things like Spinach-Pesto Lasagna and Southwest of the Border Chicken and Pollo de Grillo.

I have: six boxes of hand-me-down baby clothes. Two cribs, two Pack 'n Plays, one bouncy seat, one baby swing. Two car seats. Two hand-knit baby blankets. A dozen Avent bottles, a dozen preemie bottles, a Medela breast pump. A baby-wipes warmer and a contoured changing pad. A BabyBjörn front pack. Three dozen cloth diapers.

I have: a few pain pills, a few sleeping pills, and a prescription for Tylenol 3, all from my discharge from the hospital. I haven't used them, because I don't want any of it to reach the babies through my breast milk, especially Avery. Instead, I take regular Tylenol, and alternate with regular Motrin. I drink water by the gallon jug, which I keep in the fridge, or sometimes in the freezer, if I can remember to put it there. And half cups of coffee filled mostly with milk, gulped from my ceramic mug with violets painted on it, because even though I know coffee isn't good for breast-feeding mothers, I can't get through the day without it.

I have: a dozen phone numbers written on a sheet of yellow construction paper taped to the fridge. The direct line to the NICU, the general number for Community Medical Center, the number for St. Joseph's, the number of Dr. Rosquist's practice, the number of our family practitioner, the number of Home Healthcare for Avery's monitor. Tom's folks, my folks, Sarah, Phyllis, our neighbor Cathy, whom I still haven't spoken to. She has not called me back, and I don't think they are on vacation.

There's the number for Shodair, the children's hospital that did the genetic testing on Avery. They have a hotline for parents of children with Down syndrome. I haven't called them yet, because I don't know what to say.

There's the number of the National Down Syndrome Society (NDSS), and also the number of the National Association for Down Syndrome (NADS). A number for an organization called the Child Development Center (CDC), too, and I don't know who they are or why I have their number, but I do. It was given to me in the hospital and I was told to set up an appointment.

I have all of these things, my own support van, if you will, but I am stuck. I can't bring myself to make any calls. Every time I think of Avery's Down syndrome, I start to cry. And I can barely manage our lives as it is—someone has to keep this family afloat, and I am the only big person around. I can't allow myself the luxury of falling apart. I'm much better off thinking of him as a baby, or just as Avery. I'm getting used to simply doing what works.

With this second pregnancy, I'd dreamed of using cloth diapers for the baby. When we found out it would be two babies, I still thought I might try it. But I've let go of that idea, and use the disposables from the firemen.

I'd also wanted to breast-feed both babies. Bennett is learning, Avery is not. I'm letting go of that idea, too.

I'd thought I would have a chance to hold on to this newborn time, a second chance to experience what seemed so fleeting with Carter. I've let go of that, too.

Let go, let go, let go, and hold on for the ride.


Bennett is only content when he is snuggled in the front pack, so I wear him in the BabyBjörn a lot. He hates having his diaper changed, so we've come to a system that he tolerates: the contoured changing pad is on top of the dryer, which I turn on when he's getting changed. The wipes are in the warmer, next to the lotion, next to a stack of diapers, everything lined up in easy reach. I know this is not advised—the pad has a label warning against using it on anything but a changing table—but Bennett simply doesn't care. He hates the swing, hates the bouncy seat, and will only sleep if he's tucked snugly into his car seat.

Avery is like a big open cup. Everything that goes down tips right out if he's jostled. I call Dr. Rosquist, who calls our family practitioner, who calls me and advises me to give him Zantac. The Zantac spills out, too. So I tilt everything. I put books under the head of the crib, under two of the four Pack 'n Play legs. Or I put him in his bouncy seat, without the bouncing. Or in the swing, without the swinging. As long as he stays upright for a half hour after feeding, he seems to do okay.

In all other ways, Avery is an easy baby. He sucks on his hand and pulls his foot up to his mouth. He is trying to smile. He sleeps well, and he tolerates his monitor, which gives him that red rash, something that would send Bennett howling. He has honey-colored hair that is thick and straight; Bennett is bald. He has rosy, chubby cheeks. When he sleeps, you'd never know he has Down syndrome. He looks peaceful and perfect, like the babies in the Anne Geddes calendars.

When we found out we were having twins, Tom said he secretly wished that the babies would be as different from each other as possible. No Barry and Larry, no Anna and Hannah. I agreed. I wanted them each to be themselves, and even now, at six weeks old, I can see that we got what we hoped for. Our babies are hot and cold, salty and sweet, oil and water. They are as different as night and day.


I don't know why it's so difficult for me to ask for help, but it is. I pick up the phone, put it down. Pick it up, put it down. Up, down.

What would I say? "Help, come quick"? Or "I've fallen and I can't get up"? In my family, we were taught not to complain. My sister and I were told to be grateful for the things we had, to always "look to the sunny side of life." For us, complaining was the worst thing you could do. Instead, we'd make jokes, and try to laugh.

I dial Sarah's number. "Hey, it's me," I say.

"Hello! Good to hear from you! How are you?"

"Okay, I guess, if you consider dark circles under your eyes to be achievements. How are you?"

"Oh, stop. I'm sure you're beautiful, a radiant mother with her beautiful babies and all that. What's up?"

"Tom's out of town, and I was wondering if you'd come over and keep me company tonight. I'm getting a little nutty, and I need a grown-up to talk to. I'd love it if it could be you."

"Of course! Let me bring supper. Should I bring the kids? They'd love to see Carter."

"I have a ton of food. You don't have to cook. And definitely bring the boys. It would be wonderful to see them."

"I'm bringing supper. No discussion. When should we come?"

"Is an hour too soon?"

"No, the sooner the better. It'll do the kids good to get out of the house. See you then."

I hang up the phone. It isn't so hard, after all. I dial two more numbers: the NDSS and the NADS. I leave messages at both places, asking to be put on their mailing lists. Again, it isn't as hard as I thought it would be.

I dial one more number and leave another message. "Hi, I'm calling for Cathy. It's Jennifer. I hope you're okay. Haven't heard from you in a while. We're home, and I have some news to share. Give me a call when you get a chance."

Soon enough, I hear Sarah's white Chevy Blazer pulling up

our driveway, dust trailing behind it. Car doors open; then comes the sound of her two boys, ages four and two, hopping out. "Carter, Carter," they call. I open our front door and there she is, tall and tan, smiling her dazzling smile.

"Hello, honey," she says, and leans in and gives me a kiss on the cheek and a hug. Her arms are full of bags—more baby clothes, cold zucchini soup, French bread. Containers of macaroni and cheese for the kids, cubes of cantaloupe. And there is a bottle of verbena hand lotion for me. "For your diaper-changing hands," she says.

It's the beginning of early evening, when the sunlight slants and the mountains turn shades of orange and red. The smoke from the forest fires has thinned. We gather everyone and everything and go outside to sit on blankets on the grass.

She carries Bennett gently, tenderly, and I know how much she wishes she could have a third baby. I hold Avery, the monitor slung over my shoulder, and make a joke about how it's the newest accessory in Babyland.

"You don't have to worry about SIDS this way," I say. My jostling sets off the monitor and the joke falls flat. I can see in Sarah's eyes that the alarm has startled her, so I reset it quickly.

"It's okay," I say. "It's nothing."

We sit for a while. I'm unsure what to say. I'm afraid that my life is too much for her, for anyone, until she breaks the silence.

"I've been thinking," she says.

"Yes?"

"About Babyland. I've decided it's like this: I've made two trips to Babyland, and I consider myself very lucky."

"You are. You have two beautiful boys," I say.

"And that's enough. Really, it is," she says.

The light across the mountains shifts and changes from pink to orange. The sun is a red ball hanging over the lake. I wonder if my life has helped her reach this conclusion. When you go to

Babyland, there are no guarantees. No one expects twins, monitors with shrill alarms, Down syndrome. But this idea doesn't feel right. I think she's telling me something else.

There was a moment a few years after my first pregnancy when I found myself in the kitchen making chicken soup for a new mother, stirring the pot in front of me, watching the pieces of chicken and the disks of carrots swirl around and around, and I began crying. I couldn't help myself. I realized that I wanted to be the one whose life was too full; I wanted to be the one who didn't even have time to boil water. I wanted that feeling of the world becoming too vivid; I wanted to know that intense, all-consuming newborn love one more time. The thought seemed impossible, and I knew all the reasons why I shouldn't want it. But I did. I wanted to go to Babyland one more time, and I wanted it with a desperation that defied reason. And now, I think Sarah is telling me she knows that feeling, and that letting go of it is hard.

"Here's an idea," I say. "Maybe Babyland is never the same place twice. Maybe it's like time travel. If you go back and alter even one thing, your whole world is altered. I thought it would be more familiar, this time. But it isn't. Everything's different. I'm different, too," I say.

"Sure. There's no going back, is there?" she says.

"No. I don't think there is. Although I wish you could. But maybe with little breaks, like weekends off," I say.

"You know, I miss it," she says.

"You only think you miss it. Come over to my house more and you'll remember how much work it is."

"I remember," she says. "I remember. It feels like yesterday."

Bennett is asleep in the front pack, which Sarah is wearing. Avery is lying on a baby quilt, sucking on his fist. For a moment, through Sarah's eyes, I see my life as round and full and good, a feeling that is as surprising to me as a burst of cool air on a hot, hot summer night.

We watch the older boys play in the twilight, until their game sours. Someone has thrown dirt on someone else; there are tears and hurt feelings, and possibly someone called someone else a bad name. It's clear that it's time to split up and head our separate ways, though Sarah promises she'll drop off the boys at home with Ric and then be right back.

None of these things matter to me—though I can see that Sarah is upset that our night has not gone perfectly. How can I tell her that I'm not interested in perfect? How can I tell her that the gift she's given me is one of a normal night, complete with fusses and fights and all the things of life with small children, and that for a few hours, those few hours with her, I felt completely, exactly like my old self?

I want to say all of this and more. I want her to go to Babyland if it's what she wants, or not, if that's what she wants. I want her to be happy, and I want to be happy again, too. She's reminded me that I am grateful for my children, and for that, I am grateful for her, too.

All I can think to say is "Thank you so much. You saved my life tonight." She has known me a long time. I hope she knows how much I mean it.

# 6

### ✑

# Cathy Can't Handle Us

Y ou know crocodiles, Mommy?" asks Carter.

"Mmm, yes." I'm fumbling with the visor on the stroller, a blue-and-green InSTEP double jogger with yellow trim, which is used, but new to us.

"They poop," Carter says.

"Why, yes. Yes, they do. So do babies, and so do you."

Back at home, it seemed like a good idea to get us all outdoors for some fresh air. The sun is hot and the babies are crying and I wonder, now, what was I thinking? The double stroller has a hinky wheel that pulls to the right and Carter keeps running ahead, because he thinks he knows the way.

We're walking to Cathy's house, or rather, walking along the gravel road that leads to her house, because despite my numerous phone messages, I still haven't talked with her. I want to walk by and see if they are around. Carter is anxious to get there and play with Cathy's son, who's the same age. I'm tired of leaving phone messages and I want to see for myself if what I suspect is true. I'm thinking that, simply put, Cathy can't handle us.

When they first moved next door, I cut flowers from my garden, wrapped them in a raffia bow, took them over and introduced myself. It's been four years already. In that time, there was a broken wrist (her son) and a broken leg (my son), playdates, birthday parties, eggs and milk borrowed, cherry pies shared in a pie dish passed back and forth. When they left for the weekends, we fed their cats and watered their plants, letting ourselves in with a spare key. She wanted a flower garden, so I took plants from mine and we moved them behind her house, some of them the very plants I'd brought her flowers from years earlier. She's a woman of medicine who has training as a nurse practitioner and is the wife of a pediatrician. Her name is not really Cathy, but I will call her that, because despite everything, I feel the need to protect her.

She grew up Catholic, in a family of six children. They went to mass each Sunday in her family's lime green Volkswagen Beetle, all eight of them piled into the tiny vehicle like the clown car in a circus. When she left home, her father told her she'd never amount to much because her head was in the clouds. She'd wanted to be an artist.

On her fortieth birthday, she cried because she felt old. I baked a chocolate cake that we ate in the shade of my porch. There was a miscarriage (hers) and a pregnancy (mine). She told me she'd started taking Paxil to help with depression. Soon enough she was pregnant again, and now, after years of almost weekly conversations, she's not returning my phone calls.

Cathy's house is a big sprawling affair with huge windows that look out over the lake, set back from the road on a large grassy slope of lawn. The yard has a split-rail fence, and at the driveway, the gate is open. This is the first sign that they are home. The second clue is her Chevy Suburban parked alongside the house. These facts are undeniable and I feel a little stab in the pit of my stomach.

I consider pushing the stroller up the driveway and banging on the door. I will tell her that there's nothing to be afraid of. I'll tell her that we're not contagious—you can't catch twins, or Down syndrome. I'll show her the babies, and say, *Look! See how wonderful they are?*, which is something I want to believe, and I need to see it reflected in the eyes of the people around me, especially the people who know me best.

But she's seven months pregnant. She's trying to make sense of her life, just as I'm trying to make sense of mine. I can see how it will go. She won't answer the door. She'll twist the blinds closed and click the dead bolt until we go away.

Or worse: she will answer the door, and she'll look at me with a fake smile and an excuse about how busy she's been. She'll say how lovely the babies are, looking at Bennett while she's speaking, and not at Avery. She'll touch Bennett's cheek, coo and smile at him, and then look away, out across the lake.

I grab Carter by the hand and say, "Oh, looks like they're busy. Let's get back to our house and I'll give you a Popsicle."

He accepts my bribe and starts skipping down the road in the opposite direction. I manage to turn the stroller and its wobbly wheel and I follow him along the twisty gravel lane, back to the safety of home.

What a mess we are, my blue-eyed babies and red-eyed me. The house smells of milk and baby lotion and diapers. Avery is still hooked to his monitor, the tubes and tanks of oxygen piled in a corner of the living room near the couch, in case we need them. And Bennett cries inconsolably most of the time. I can't remember when I've slept for more than an hour at a stretch.

In the packet of information we got from the NICU, there is a photocopy about what to expect with preemies. It says that babies who are born early may prefer to sleep with the lights on, having grown accustomed to it in the NICU. They may need background noise to stay asleep; again, like in the NICU. They may have grown used to the NICU schedule, which parents should try to maintain at home. The photocopy also says that preemies may have sensitive nervous systems, and might respond harshly to any extra sensory stimulus.

Babies born prematurely are "at risk" for a number of things, including improper attachment, sensory integration issues, and gross motor development delays. They should also have their vision and hearing monitored, and parents should be especially careful of a flu-like virus called RSV. Preemies have what is called an adjusted age, which reflects not their actual age in weeks or months but their age as if they were born on their original due date. The "at risk" description and the adjusted age applies throughout the first two years of life.

So far, Bennett is unlike any baby I've known. He cries almost constantly; what varies is the intensity of his cries. He hates the sun. He hates fresh air. Even the slightest breeze brushing across his cheek annoys him. He dislikes having his diaper changed, he dislikes having his clothes off. He hates music, and yet he doesn't seem to mind the sound of Avery's monitor going off, or the ringing of the phone.

These are the things he likes: breast-feeding, being carried in the front pack, sleeping on his stomach with his knees drawn up into him; and Avery. He loves Avery. If I put them in the crib together, Bennett sidles up to Avery and pushes against him. Avery moves away, and Bennett sidles some more, and Avery inches away some more, until Avery's wires twist loose and his alarm goes off.

The beeping doesn't bother either of the babies, but it bothers me. My heart leaps, and wherever I am in the house, whatever it is that I'm doing, I stop and rush to check the monitor. If it were a real alarm, this is what I'm supposed to do: stim Avery, which means revive him by tickling his feet, or blowing in his face, or touching his cheek, or hands, or feet. If these things don't snap him out of it, increase the intensity. Clap loudly, yell. Then the hardcore measures: quickly attach the nasal cannula to the oxygen, wave it below his nose, and if that doesn't work, put the cannula directly in his nostrils. Check his pulse. Begin infant CPR. Call for help.

I don't let myself think about the extremes too much; if I do, it makes me sick to my stomach. I think instead about breathing—deep, full, rhythmic breaths. Mine, and Avery's. Together, like I did in the hospital, as if my will, my desire, could be enough for both of us. It's become the cadence of our lives, the steady breathing in and out, and it's always there, and I'm always thinking of it, even when sleeping, even in my dreams.

I've reached a new state of exhaustion. I think Bennett might have colic, but it's hard to unravel his mysterious crying when simple tasks, such as putting each shoe on the correct foot, seem nearly impossible. And in the midst of the sleep deprivation, I'm trying to untangle the mystery of the papers given to us by a social worker at the hospital for SSI and Medicaid. The forms need to be filled out in order to see if we qualify for either of these services, but I'm so tired that my brain isn't working right.

The papers have the same governmental flair as the forms for income taxes, only these are worse. If I fill them out and we do qualify for aid, we will have become, officially, "the needy" that I've spent my life donating to or collecting for, and my pride is a hard, stale cookie to swallow. If we don't qualify, I've wasted three or more precious hours, which is unforgivable to a woman so desperate for sleep.

The first form is the SSA-3820-BK Disability Report—Child, which asks for detailed medical records, with graphs and subsections that tend to blur if I stare at them too long. I can manage sections one, two, four, five, six, seven, eight, nine, and ten. It's section three, "The child's illnesses, injuries, or conditions and how they affect him/her," that stops me. I can't bring myself to fill it out. It's contrary to every wish I have for the babies, every good hope that I am trying to hold on to for them.

For Avery: He has trisomy 21 and we don't know how it will affect his development and we won't know what this will mean to him until he is much older. We love him and are going to accept and encourage him and we'll see where that gets us.

For Bennett: He is a premature newborn at risk for a number of things, but I think with love and consistency he will outgrow it. It's good that we have two babies—each one needs the other and together, with patience and guidance, they will find their way.

Or another version, with a darker slant: Avery has Down syndrome. He is having reflux issues and is on a home monitor, for an undetermined length of time, due to periodic episodes of apnea and bradycardia. Bennett is hyperstimulated, is having difficulty with attachment, and is showing symptoms of failure to thrive. I am the new mother of twins, caring for the babies plus another child, who is just four years old, at the very end of a twisty gravel road deep in the woods, far from the hospital and its support.

I can't write it. I won't even think it, much less put it there on the page in ink, so permanent. It feels like a death sentence.

The second form is the SSA-3375-BK Function Report. In it, I'm supposed to list the things the babies should be doing but aren't. I can't fill this one out, either, for the same reasons. The third is the Authorization to Disclose Information to the Social Security Administration (SSA), which is simple, basic information, only I have to fill out and sign ten copies of it, five for each baby (no photocopies). If I were in a better frame of mind, it would be laughable—one of the pages I have to sign is my acknowledgment that all of this paperwork, which is more than I had to fill out when we bought our house, is in compliance with the Paperwork Reduction Act.

The forms are meant to determine if either of the babies qualifies for SSI, as best as I can tell. SSI is supplemental income, which sometimes includes food stamps and Medicaid. Rules for getting SSI vary from state to state, and the amount offered also varies. I go to Social Security's Web site, and only become more confused. It says that a family may not own more than $3,000 worth of items, but certain things don't count. A home is not counted, for example, or one car. A burial plot doesn't count, or up to $3,000 in burial funds. But we have a second car. Tom's truck is worth more than $3,000. I call the toll-free number and learn that we will not qualify for SSI or Medicaid, or any of it, because of the truck. Why didn't someone say so right up front? A simple question: Do you have two cars? Or even, do you have $3,000 in assets? Okay, then, move on down the line, lady, we can't help you here.

I pull the papers together, shove them back in their manila envelope, and set it on top of the bookshelf, with all the other paperwork. I don't know if this news makes me happy or sad. It's good to appreciate how much we have; but I was counting on some help—I was hoping, at least, for better insurance. We can't continue our coverage, a major-medical family plan with a $5,000 deductible at $526 a month, for much longer. And I wonder if we go off the insurance, will we be able to reinsure Avery, or any of us, later?

There are other bits of business that I've been avoiding. On the bookshelf, near the SSA papers and the book *Babies with Down Syndrome*, is an order form for birth announcements. The babies are home. They are almost three months old. And aside from the phone calls that Tom made from the hospital, and the calls we hoped other people would make for us, we haven't announced ourselves, our new arrivals, to anyone.

When Carter was born, we ordered cards from a company that specialized in baby announcements. The card was blue and had all the important information: name, date of birth, length, weight. Tucked inside the little card, we included a copy of the newborn photo taken at the hospital. We intended to do the same thing for our second pregnancy, only our good intentions had gotten derailed, for the same reasons I was having difficulty filling out all the SSA forms. We found a place that had a card for twins; one birth date, but two spaces for names, two spaces for measurements. But there are no spaces for "number of weeks premature," no boxes to check for "number of chromosomes." Our story doesn't fit the blanks, and it seems dishonest to me to leave out what feels like the most important details.

Tom and I have circular discussions about it, round conversations with no beginning and no end that pick up apropos of nothing, and end for no apparent reason, only to be started again later. In the middle of changing a diaper, I suggest, "We could do a letter. Like a Christmas letter, only a summertime one. And then we could explain."

"Explain what?" Tom asks. "What's there to explain? We have two babies, they are home, that's our news. The people who know us, the people who are part of our lives, already know the rest. The ones who don't know, well, maybe there's a reason for that. Maybe that's okay."

"What about a photo?" I begin, while emptying the dishwasher. "All we have are those horrid ones from the NICU. They look so scary. Or now. With Bennett crying all the time and Avery still attached to the monitor. What do we do about a photo?"

"No photo" is Tom's answer. But again, I hesitate. It seems as if we are hiding something, and I'm not sure I want to hide.

"We could do a little movie, a digital home movie, and send it out over the Internet," I say over coffee. But as soon as I suggest it, I know it's a bust. Neither of us can do that, and even if we could, about half of our relatives wouldn't be able to open it. I could easily imagine the confusion we would cause, and the frustration.

Our answer, for the time being, is to do nothing by default.


The question of the announcements is revisited in a dozen small ways: at the grocery store, when the checkout lady notices I'm no longer pregnant and asks after the babies; at the mailbox, while chatting with the mailman; at the door, when the UPS delivery man needs a signature. All simple questions—"How are the babies?" or "How's the family?" or "How are you?"—with any number of possible answers. Which version is the truth?

I find myself dumbstruck quite often, nodding and smiling mutely, completely at a loss for words. Again, Tom and I have rolling, rambling conversations about what we should do.

"I saw Mike at the post office," he begins.

"Did you tell him?"

"Sort of. I tried to. It was busy, and we were in line, and people were listening. I told him the babies had some health concerns, but that we were all home and doing fine."

Or, me. "I tried to call Cathy again. I told her I had a nice cherry pie over here and that she should call me if she was around."

"Why do you care? Let it go. If she can't handle us, it's her problem. Besides, it's better that we know now, right up front, what her feelings are," he says.

"That's just it. I don't know what her feelings are. We haven't ever talked about it," I say.

"I think she's made it pretty clear. You know, a person can say a lot without using any words at all."

At what point do you let go? At what point do you stop trying? I've never been good at recognizing that moment. When I phone someone, I let it ring and ring, certain that if I only hold on a bit longer, *that* will be the ring that is answered.

I call Sarah instead.

"Hi, it's me," I say. "She's still not answering."

"Did you leave a message?" Sarah asks.

"Yes. But I know she's home."

"Are you sure?"

"The car is in the driveway," I answer.

"What are you going to do? I mean, this is all so bizarre. It doesn't make sense," Sarah says.

"Have you heard how she is?" I ask.

"I think she's having trouble with the pregnancy. Not that the baby is in danger, but that she's having a hard time. She's been sick a lot, and she's been feeling really tired," Sarah says.

"Is it a boy or a girl?"

"It's a girl," she says. "They went to Great Falls to have the 3-D ultrasound. I don't want to upset you, but they were looking specifically for signs of Down syndrome. The AFP came back fine, but she was still worried about it."

"Of course," I say.

"Are you okay?" she asks.

"Yes, I'm fine."

"I wasn't going to say anything. But you asked."

"No, it's okay. And I did. I asked. I guess I have my answer," I say.

"If that's it, then you're better off anyway," Sarah says.

"I know," I say. "I know."


I call Phyllis.

"Hey, it's me. Is this a good time?" I ask.

"Of course, what's up?"

"I need advice. How do you know when it's time to let go of something?"

"Like what?" she asks.

"A friendship," I say.

"You're not talking about me, I hope."

"Of course not! It's complicated. Look, what are you doing now? Can I come over for a minute? I'll tell you in person."

"Okay, then. I'll see you soon."

I pack up the freshly fed, freshly burped babies, in fresh diapers and fresh clothes. I put a little hat on each one—an acorn hat for Avery with a little knob on top, a blue cap for Bennett that matches his eyes. Each into his car seat, each into the car. Then Carter—shorts and a clean shirt, shoes. I grab a sippy of water for him and a clear plastic bottle of water for me, for the ride to town.

Phyllis lives on its outskirts, in a light blue house with lighter blue trim. Her yard is shady and green and dotted with trees—a big old willow for climbing; cherry and pear trees; hybrid poplars that rustle in the breeze. A row of lilacs bloom along one side of the fenced yard and raised beds line another, where Phyllis grows beans and peas and strawberries and flowers.

When I pull into the driveway, she is already outside on her porch swing, waiting. My three passengers have fallen asleep. I motion to her, using the universal sign for nighty night—hands folded together brought to the cheek, head tilted, eyes closed. She waves at me to stay in the car, and comes over. I tell her about the phone messages.

"What would you do, if you were me?" I ask.

"I'd probably bake her something," she says.

"Did it. I offered pie. Who can say no to pie?" I ask.

"No one," she says.

"I'm about done trying," I say.

"Sure," she says. "No one can blame you."

"I feel so sad," I say. "If I could only talk to her about it."

"But she doesn't want to talk to you, and it takes two to make a conversation. Maybe she'll come around. Give it time. That's what I'd do. I'd give it time."

"Time," I repeat. "I'll try it, I guess. It's the only thing I haven't done."

"I have something of my own to tell you," she says.

"Uh-oh, it sounds serious. What's going on?"

"I'm pregnant," she says.

"Oh, my heavens. Are you okay?" I ask.

"Yes, I'm fine. A little in shock. But I'm fine."

"What can I do? Is there anything you need?" I ask.

"Seeing you is enough. I was really worried about you," she says. Her voice breaks, and I can see her eyes have tears in them. I glance back at the babies, asleep in their little hats. Avery's has tilted down over one eye, spry, my brave acorn. I feel the rawness of it all, my news, and hers. Life. I begin to cry, too.

"Are yours happy tears," I ask, "or sad?"

"Not-afraid tears," she says.

"Why?" I ask.

"You," she says.

"Me? Why me?" I ask.

"You can handle it. Now that I see you, I know you can handle it."

"Oh, I doubt it," I say. I think about what I've said, and I say it again. "Oh, I really doubt it. You know me. I'm a doubter!"

We begin laughing, crying and laughing at the same time. It's an old conversation: Phyllis has faith, I have doubt. She reaches in and gives me a hug. We stay like this for a while. I feel uneasy leaving her. Five children, and a baby on the way. My kindhearted friend.

"Will you be okay?" I ask again.

"Yes. I feel like this baby is one bright spot in a long season of gray."

Babies tuck in around our lives, like water. I can barely remember my life before Carter; soon I won't be able to remember life before the twins. Avery is awake now and is softly sucking his hand. Big blue eyes watching me. He is the happiest baby. I think I'll start sucking my hand. Maybe it will help.

The books I ordered are waiting at the mailbox for me when we return home. I unwrap the package to the Kelly green cover of *Understanding Down Syndrome: An Introduction for Parents*, by Cliff Cunningham, and the mostly yellow cover of *A Parent's Guide to Down Syndrome: Toward a Brighter Future*, by Siegfried M. Pueschel. I thumb the pages. The green book has a detailed table of contents that already seems too complicated. I flip through it until I reach the end, where an appendix of black-and-white photographs catches my eye. Each page shows one child, through the years. A baby sleeping on a father's chest. First steps with a train-engine push toy. A birthday party with cake and pointed hats. Splashing in a blue plastic swimming pool. Banging on pots and pans. Making a gingerbread house. A school day, with a backpack in front of the school bus. Soccer. T-ball. Everyone is smiling and happy and a feeling of nostalgia comes over me, one I get every time I see collections of family photos. Here are whole lives, lived.

I set the green book back in the box and take out the yellow one by Siegfried M. Pueschel, a name I recognize from the Web sites. Dr. Pueschel is a professor, an advocate, and a parent of a son with Down syndrome. His book's table of contents lists twenty-four chapters, which seems like a lot. I scan them, and notice the first ten apply to Avery; the rest deal with older children.

*So,* I think, *it's about two hundred pages of reading for the green book, and two hundred more for the yellow.* My brain hurts just imagining the extra work, but I can't ignore the books now that they're here. I won't know what's in them, and learn if it's helpful or not, until I begin reading.

When Carter was little, he used to eat books. He'd lick the pages, chew on the corners, and sometimes I'd find a wadded-up piece of a page in his tiny mouth. I wish I could do that now—I wish I could devour these books, ingest them, eat them all up in one sitting. It becomes clear to me that I need a completely different kind of book—I need a CliffsNotes version of these books, I need a quick outline of what to get where and when. Now that I'm in Holland, I need a road map.

When I was in college, I had trouble managing my time. I'd begin the semester with good intentions, but before I knew it, finals week was upon me and my mountain of unread books. I'd plow through the information in a mad rush, feeling guilty—it seemed like a very poor way to learn about subjects I professed to love.

But now, I'm grateful for all that experience cramming. I put on a pot of coffee, I feed and bathe Carter and the babies, put them to bed, and I begin. The green book is first, *Understanding Down Syndrome: An Introduction for Parents,* by Cliff Cunningham, because of the photos in the back. I look at them more closely, trying to find a child who reminds me of Avery. I don't succeed. I try to look for parents who look like me, or Tom. Siblings like Carter, or Carter's age. Again, nothing. The book was first published in 1982, and everything looks dated. I'm reminded of high school; I was a sophomore then. I'd just gotten my driver's license; after school, I worked at the local grocery store as a checkout clerk. The girl I was then; the mother I am now. I imagine my own page of photos; a life, passing. But I'm getting distracted. I turn to the table of contents.

Chapter one is titled "Will We Cope? What Are They Like?" I skip it. I don't have any choice but to cope. Chapter two is "Feelings and Emotions." Again, skip it, no time. Chapter three, "What Effects Will It Have on the Family?" Skip. And I'm beginning to become annoyed. This all seems very negative to me. I don't appreciate the doom and gloom. Chapter four is about what causes Down syndrome, which I believe I understand already. Five is about physical and medical characteristics; six is personality and temperament; seven is "Mental, Motor and Social Development." I return to five.

It begins with a warning in bold type: the chapter discusses all characteristics associated with Down syndrome, but the majority of children with DS will have only a small number of them. Care should be taken when relating this information to your baby or child.

*Interesting,* I think.

And on the next page, I see more words in bold, "People with Down syndrome have far more 'normal' than 'abnormal' characteristics. You should try to keep this in mind when you read this chapter, because I will mainly be writing about what is different from the 'norm.'"

*Even more interesting.* I skim through the chapter, and read closely the physical characteristics of babies with Down syndrome. Avery has about half of them. I learn that the stars in his eyes have a name—Brushfield spots. I learn that his button nose, and tiny ears, are common, as is his crooked pinky finger. It's likely that he'll grow more slowly than Bennett, and have a smaller head circumference, shorter arms, and shorter legs.

I continue reading, paying particular attention to the section on hearing. I learn that 80–90 percent of children with DS will have some hearing loss in one or both ears. The loss is temporary, often due to fluid, and is unlikely to hinder the child, which makes me feel hopeful about Avery's left ear. The section stresses the importance of regular testing, and I feel the pinch of guilt—I need to reschedule his hearing test.

I discover other, various things: Avery's teeth will probably come in late, and in an unusual order; children with DS tend to have looser muscles than other children and are floppier; many people with Down syndrome are particularly fond of swimming, as it supports their loose-jointedness; Avery might have poorer circulation than Bennett and I should pay attention to keeping his hands and feet warm.

I also discover that each chapter in the green book has a summary section at the end, which is extremely helpful. I read all of the summaries of all the chapters. I also notice that in back there's a detailed resource section. Despite my early misgivings, I like this book very much. It has potential. I set it aside and plan to read it again, cover to cover, when I have more time. I turn my attention toward Dr. Pueschel's yellow book.

Bennett is awake and I go to him, book in hand. I settle him and me in the green rocking chair and he nurses and falls back asleep. I don't dare move, for fear that I'll wake him. The only light comes into the room from the hallway, but it's the best I can manage; at least for a little while, I have an opportunity, so I take it.

Dr. Pueschel's book is a collection of essays, some of them written by him, some written by others. The first chapter is called "From Parent to Parent," which isn't written by the doctor, so I skip it. Same with the second chapter, and the third, which is called "Raising a Child with a Handicap." The word "handicap" troubles me; I know from my People First Language that it's outdated. I begin with chapter four, which is the first chapter written by Dr. Pueschel, called "A Historical Viewpoint."

I'd never considered the historical context of Down syndrome before, but of course there is one. The earliest evidence is a Saxon skull dating back to the seventh century that has structural changes seen in children with DS. Pictorially, the facial features of sculptures from the Olmec culture three thousand years ago resemble people with DS. There are fifteenth-century artists whose paintings seem to depict babies with DS, and in the dim half-light coming from the hallway, I can see the resemblance. It gives me comfort, thinking of our family, of Avery, as part of the greater history of humankind.

Bennett is stirring, so I switch sides, settle him again, then resume skimming the book with urgency, looking through the pages for anything new or different, because I sense that my window of opportunity is coming to a close. I see the squiggly lines of more karyotypes; my eyes rest on chromosome number 21. Always, three. They remind me of ellipses, *dot dot dot.*

I skip the chapter on prenatal diagnosis—what use is that to us?—and move on to the next, about physical characteristics. I recognize many of the terms from my earlier reading: Brushfield spots, epicanthic fold, helix, palate. This chapter, too, stresses that no child will have every characteristic, and urges physicians not to overemphasize physical traits, but instead to look at the baby as a human being deserving of nurturing and love.

I continue scanning and skimming until I reach chapter ten, which is my cutoff. Here, I notice that the discussion turns toward early developmental stimulation, and something called Early Intervention, which sounds familiar. I make a note to read more of this book later. For tonight, I'm done. I gently stand, still carrying Bennett. I make my way through the house, turning out the lights. Bennett's eyes flutter in his sleep; he's dreaming. I put him in the swing and wake Avery for his bottle, which I feed him in the crook of my arm, marveling at this little baby as if we'd just met.

"We should send out the announcements," I tell Tom.

"Okay," he says. "Which ones?"

"The ones we chose before the babies came. The one with the pea pod on it, the two peas in a pod."

"Okay," he says. "Fine by me."

"I want you to do it, though. Go online and order them. We have the babies, they are home, and that's enough. You were right. The rest of it, if people don't already know, it's no one's concern," I say.

"What made you change your mind?" he asks.

"I'm sick of thinking about it. And I don't want to do nothing. It's time," I say.

"What about the photo?"

"I'll take a photo. Whatever I get will be fine," I say.

"Are you sure about this?"

"Yes."

We include the birth date, and each baby's name and measurements. No letter, no witty comments about bonus chromosomes or designer genes. A photo of the babies in little white outfits, Avery's wires hidden under his shirt, Bennett's face blotchy and red from crying. Our two peas in a pod, as different as could be, yet bound together by one simple word: family. Welcome to the family. You belong to us and we belong to you. Everything that needs to be said isn't even on the card; it isn't said with words at all, but with action. Licking the last envelope closed, writing the final address on the front, putting the very last postage stamp in the corner, it all feels like a great accomplishment.

And Tom and I finally come up with rules for telling people. We decide that there is one simple way to know what to say: consider the spirit in which the question is asked. Take, for example, the ubiquitous "How's it going?" No one really expects an answer; it's another way of saying, "Hey." Along these same lines, some questions are not really asking for answers. So, "How're the babies?" if said in a light, conversational way, might be answered with, "Great! We love being out of the NICU." Which is true, and is what I say to the lady behind the counter in the post office when I deliver the bundles of announcements.

Or, "How *are* the babies?" if asked in a more serious tone by a close friend, might be answered with a longer, more detailed response. Which is what Tom chooses when Scott, his friend since kindergarten, calls. Tom takes the phone into the bedroom and disappears for an hour, which seems like a very short amount of time, considering all that's happened in the last three months.

And to the question of whom we should tell, we decide this: tell anyone you want, any time you want, only if you want. It's nobody's business, really. I don't go around telling everyone that I was born with an astigmatism, though I imagine when I'm wearing my glasses people might assume something is wrong with my vision. If they want to know more, they can ask me. And if I want to talk about it, I will. If not, I won't. It's that simple.

Finally, there's Cathy. I try calling one more time, and get the machine.

"Hi, it's Jennifer. I'm not going to call anymore. If you want to get ahold of me, you know the number. Call anytime. If not, just know that we're home, and we're okay, and I wish you the same. I hope you're doing well. That's it. That's all I wanted to say."

I didn't know it then, but it was the last time I'd call that house. In the fall, she had her baby, a healthy little girl. In the winter, they posted a FOR SALE BY OWNER sign on the wood fence around their yard. In the summer, the house sold, and they moved to town. I don't have her new phone number.

I see her sometimes, at the park or the grocery store, and though we are both cordial, we never speak of what's passed between us, so that now, it all seems like a dream. I knew a woman, once, in this dream, and her name wasn't Cathy, but I'll call her that, because even now, I miss her.

# 7

❧

# They All Do That

Tom and I bundle up everyone and drive through the fall sunshine. The breeze has a coolness that tells me summer is over and the air smells like smoke, only not from the forest fires, but from chimneys and woodstoves. The leaves on the aspens have begun to yellow, and the needles on the larch are turning bright orange, the color of pumpkins.

There are so many things I don't know about how to be Avery's mom. Like the chain of his DNA, the list would reach the moon. Does he need a special team, for example? There are children's hospitals and research facilities with doctors who see only children with Down syndrome. But we live out in the woods, far from even a regular doctor. The nearest NICU is Missoula; the closest choices for big-city hospitals are Seattle or Salt Lake City, five hundred or six hundred miles away.

I asked the pediatrician from the NICU, the lemon sherbet doctor named Jennifer, what her thoughts were about Avery's care. She said that it was a matter of personal choice. She has a number of children in her practice that have Down syndrome; she also knows of several parents who prefer to take their children to the larger facilities in the cities. I'm sure her point would make perfect sense to anyone but me—I was looking for a more definitive answer. It reminded me of the early days of Avery's diagnosis. I kept asking, "But, what does it mean, what does it mean?" like the nursery rhyme: *The sky is falling, the sky is falling—what does it mean, what does it mean?*

I researched doctors and hospitals online and found the Web site of Dr. Len Leshin, a pediatrician and father of two boys, one with Down syndrome, where he's listed dozens of "Featured Abstracts About Down Syndrome." I didn't see anything that indicated the need for specialty clinic care.

Tom and I talked it over, too, taking a historic approach: What have we needed medical help with in the past? A broken leg. The occasional cold. Once, a diaper rash that wouldn't go away. All of these things were relatively minor—and if Avery was going to be like other children, mostly, then why would we travel hours and hours to see a specialist? We decided that we needed someone as close as possible, someone who knew us and our family, someone who could help with the everyday medical concerns of raising children, and that perhaps, in time, if Avery needed more care, then we would find it.

We discussed it with our family practitioner, who's been our primary care physician for almost as long as Carter has been alive. He stayed with us in the ER one long night when we all had un-explainable stomach cramps; he came in when we brought Carter to the orthopedic surgeon for X-rays. He's listened to my every concern about vaccines; he helped me recover from my first preg-nancy and helped me choose an ob-gyn for my second pregnancy. He'd even planned to be present at the delivery, something that didn't happen because of our unexpected trip to Missoula. He's taken care of our family for a long time, and he felt confident that he could help us with Avery, which made me feel confident, too.


Our doctor's office is in town next to the hospital. We are the first appointment of the day, and we've been given two time slots, so we can go over all the details of each baby's NICU stay. The wait-ing room is quiet, the receptionist sleepy and sipping coffee from a cup. Tom and the babies and Carter wait near the door while I go to the front desk. As I begin to speak, Avery's monitor goes off, sounding its single shrill note. The receptionist's eyes grow big. Tom quickly resets the alarm and I explain that it happens when Avery moves. He's okay.

"How do you live with that thing?" she asks. I don't have an answer—it's become part of everyday life, and we've never known Avery without it. I shrug. "You get used to it, I guess."

The benefit of having twins and preemies and one baby on a monitor that goes off without warning is that no one keeps you waiting. I sign release forms and make sure the insurance cards are on file; then we're quickly ushered into an exam room. Our doctor comes in a few minutes later.

He's thin and tanned from the many hours he spends outdoors, kayaking or bicycling. His eyes crinkle when he smiles and he speaks gently and softly, almost in a whisper. He's wearing an oxford cloth button-down shirt and baggy chinos. Around his neck, fastened to a thin multicolored cord that looks Mexican or Guatemalan, is a key.

In his arms are two manila file folders: one for Bennett, one for Avery. Only instead of reading AVERY, the name typed on the label is EVERY. A simple typo, one that I don't mention. It reminds me of Avery's trisomy, present in every cell of his body.

"How are you both doing?" he asks Tom and me right away, even before he looks at the babies.

I glance over to Tom to see if he will answer for us, but he nods at me to go first.

"We're doing good," I say, "fine. I mean, we're tired. But I think we're okay." Even as I say this I'm surprised—it feels true. We do seem to be okay, most days.

"Do you have enough help?" he asks me.

"Oh, yes. Tom's folks have been helping, and our friends, and we have more visitors planned. Everyone has been wonderful," I say. Again, it feels true.

"Are you managing okay?" He turns to Tom.

"Yes, we're doing good. Jen works so hard. And my parents have been out twice. We could use more sleep, sure, but otherwise we're good."

"Okay, then. I wanted to be sure. I've been in contact with the doctors down in Missoula. You've been in my heart space." I look at Tom, who hides a smile. Our doctor says things like "heart space" and means it, which is one of the reasons we like him.

The small talk over, he checks the babies, looking in their eyes, their ears. He feels their tummies, their sides, their scrotums. He listens to their hearts. He pulls their legs together and looks at knees, then feels the soles of their feet, all the while nodding to himself and making notes in their folders. I notice he takes greater care with Avery, handling him more gently, and this bothers me. I want him to treat the babies exactly the same.

When he's finished, we talk about vaccinations. With Carter, we followed the recommended schedule. But since then, I've come to know many women who feel this schedule puts too great a demand on a baby's developing immune system. Some of my friends have even chosen not to vaccinate. The books and the information on Dr. Leshin's Web site recommend following the regular vaccination schedule for Avery, but I'm uncomfortable with this plan. I feel the babies are still recovering from their early birth, and I don't want to introduce anything more to their systems. And I also feel that they've been poked and prodded enough to last a lifetime.

Our doctor listens to my concerns, as is his way. He's always listened to my opinions about our family's health, which I appreciate. Then he suggests we wait a while to begin the series of vaccinations, and proceed at a slower, gentler pace. It's an idea I can live with, and I agree to the plan. It will mean scheduling extra appointments, which might be inconvenient, but there's also the option of having the vaccinations given through the county health nurse. I promise to look into it.

We move on to the specifics of the exam. I have a little note-book in which I write all my questions, so I won't forget to ask them, and then I write the answers, so I won't forget those either. Most of my questions are about Bennett, but our doctor wants to talk about Avery first. My questions for him read: bump, hips, spit-up through nose? And my notes: "weight 10# 9 oz. 21½, bump okay, hips flexible but fine, spit-up okay, will outgrow." We go over Avery's failed hearing test, which needs to be redone. The doc makes a note to schedule an ABR (Auditory Brainstem Response) for us, which means another trip to Missoula. And then it's time to talk about the monitor.

"I see no reason to keep him on it," he tells us. "Avery's doing fine."

Tom and I exchange glances. No monitor? We'd grown accustomed to it. I think we both thought Avery would have a monitor forever. Taking him off it seems a bit scary, like taking the training wheels off a bicycle for the first time.

"Are you sure?" Tom asks.

"I mean, it's no trouble," I add. "Really. We don't mind it at all."

"I see. You think you need it. But you don't. There's no medical reason to keep him on it," he says, removing the electrodes from Avery's little chest even as he speaks. Avery grimaces, and tries to roll away.

"Look at that. He's trying to roll!" I say, proudly. "He's even doing more than Bennett. It's amazing."

I turn to Tom, who nods his approval. I look at the doctor, expecting him to agree and offer some ex-hippie wisdom, like how it's the nature of a baby to be a baby, or about how everything is beautiful in its own way. I smile in anticipation.

"They all do that, in the beginning," he says, instead. "They almost always start out ahead, but eventually, they fall behind." He adds, almost as an afterthought, "Your heart will break and break and break again."

Once more, I am stunned to silence. It feels as if I've been slapped across the face. One cold, hard smack. "They." Avery had turned into a "they." What I'd mistaken for kindness was pity. He pitied us.

Was this how it would be? Never knowing where you really stood with people? Having them ask you questions, and you answer as truthfully as you can, but they don't hear you? They assume you are being brave, or that you are in denial. They know your life better than you do, and they want no part of it. They don't even want to listen when you talk about it.

I have so much to say to our doctor that I don't know where to begin, which is becoming familiar territory to me. I'm the woman who thinks of a million witty comments after the moment has passed; the person who replays conversations in her head and alters them so that she always has the perfect last word.

We rush through the rest of the exam. My questions for Bennett read, "gassiness, diet, colic?" The answers are: weight 11# 10½ oz. 22½, possible umbilical hernia? We leave in a tumble of babies and baby carriers and me asking Carter to "hold hands."

As we pass by the receptionist, she says, "Life's sandpaper."

"Excuse me?" I ask, unsure of what I heard.

"Kids," she says. "They're life's sandpaper." She nods, knowingly.

Life is life's sandpaper, I decide on the drive home.

Both babies fall asleep quickly, and soon enough Carter is asleep, too. The road is the same one we traveled a few hours earlier; the colors of the trees are the same, the breeze is still at once sweet and bitter. Nothing has changed. All that has happened is that I'm a little more worn down.

First, I think we will leave our family doctor and find another caregiver. We will "break up" with him. It feels good to think of it. I might even write a letter, in which I tell him how insensitive he is. I'll tell him that his obsession with perfection is unhealthy and that it shouldn't be transferred onto a tiny little baby. I'll tell him that I didn't like the way he touched Avery, as if he were made of glass, and that I noticed that he said, "Ah goo" to Bennett, and not to Avery.

A little later, I remember the heart space. And the night in the ER, and the X-rays—all the years of care. I don't want to be the mother who is angry. I don't want to be the mother on the lookout for slights and injustices. I don't want to lose any more of the relationships in our lives because of Down syndrome. I believe he is a good doctor, he's the best in our small town, and I want him to care for my children. I decide to turn the proverbial other cheek, for the sake of my family.

A little later still, I think of it like this: I will not leave. Avery and I will show him another way. Avery and I will soften him. We will be life's sandpaper.


In the mailbox, a manila envelope waits for me, only I don't know that yet. I'm getting the babies up from their naps, and we're going to take a walk down to the mailbox to get the mail.

Bennett is fussy, his usual state, especially after waking. I change his diaper and let him nurse, while Avery practices his rolling on the floor. He wriggles and squirms until his whole body shakes, kind of a supercharged force of effort. He rocks back and forth until he tires; then he settles, and sucks his fist.

When Bennett is finished, I feed Avery a bottle. I've given up trying to breast-feed him, and I tell myself that it's okay because he loves his bottle, and can almost hold it with his two chubby hands. When he's done, I zip him into his pumpkin sack, a gift from my mother, and strap him upright into the double jogger stroller. I zip Bennett into his matching pumpkin sack and buckle him in, too. Then I go back inside to round up two matching shoes for Carter, and two matching shoes for me, which always seems to take longer than it should, and we're off.

It's the first time I've been outside all day, and the air feels fresh and good. The forest fires are still burning outside one of the historic lodges in Glacier National Park, and the long-term forecast is that it will take an act of nature (snow) to put them out completely. But I can smell snow in the air today—the cold sharp tang to the wind that comes down from Canada. It won't be long.

As we make our way down the winding gravel road, Carter drags a stick behind him, leaving a long, single line. "Look, Mommy, I'm making tracks. What kind of animal do you think would make this track?" he asks.

"An animal with two legs and two arms that likes to drink chocolate milk," I say.

"What kind of animal is that, Mommy?"

"A Carter," I say. He laughs at my silliness and skips away, stick still in hand, until we reach the mailbox.

Inside, the thick envelope waits for me. It's from the NDSS. I tear it open right there on the road, to reveal a dark blue folder. On its cover is a picture of a breathtakingly beautiful child—curly blond hair, big blue eyes with sparkles in the irises, chubby pink cheeks. In her hair is a yellow flower and she's sucking on her fist, just like Avery does. Beneath her are the words "A Promising Future Together: A Guide for New and Expectant Parents."

I open the folder and begin reading. "Dear Friend," starts a letter from Elizabeth Goodwin, the mother of a daughter with Down syndrome and the founder of the NDSS. I continue, and my breath catches at phrases like "reassurance," and "up-to-date information" and "congratulations." I also see "challenges," as well as "an exciting journey lies ahead." My heart beats a little bit faster—this seems to be exactly what I've been searching for. I turn the hinky stroller around and rush back to the house.

I put on a *Sesame Street* video for Carter, settle the babies on the floor, and return to the brochure. The first page is about Down syndrome, and the science of it. I see more beautiful photos, and information on prenatal tests and newborn diagnosis. The facts are all familiar to me by now; what I'm responding to is the presentation—the images of the children, happy and healthy; the good writing; the high-quality printing and photography.

Bennett is fussing, so I nurse him. I ask Carter to go to the fridge and get a bottle for Avery, and a chocolate milk for himself. I position Avery in the crook of my knee, Bennett in my arm, and the brochure on the floor beside me, and continue. I'm like a starving woman eating bread—I want more and more and more. I can't put the brochure down. I read all thirty-eight pages straight through, from "A Healthy Start" to "Early Intervention" and "Finding Support" and "Caring for Your Family" to the end, "A Promising Future." The information is not overwhelming. The language is clear and supportive, without being sentimental. It feels levelheaded and sensible—it even makes having a child with Down syndrome seem desirable.

A pocket in the back of the packet holds five laminated cards, titled "Down Syndrome Health Care Guidelines," each for a different age range, and on them is the information I need to make sure Avery receives good care. I love the laminate on the cards—to me, it shows an understanding of what life with little kids is really like. And best of all, on page seventeen, I see a photo of a little boy who is the spitting image of Avery.

I disengage myself from the babies and change them into fresh diapers. I kiss Carter on top of the head.

"What was that for, Mommy?" he asks.

"I love you, that's all," I say.

"I love you, too, and I love my daddy, and I love my brothers. I love everyone," he says happily.

"Me, too," I say. I feel something I haven't in a long while: confidence.


Avery and I are in the chapel. It's a small room toward the back of the hospital in Missoula, reached by following a labyrinth of hallways. Despite all the weeks we spent here, I didn't know this room existed until now.

The floor is covered in low-pile beige carpeting. A dieffenbachia and a fern and a spider plant, all too green to be real, are clustered in one corner. Two rows of beige stacking chairs face the front of the room, where a cross might hang. Instead, there's a plastic, lighted box. On the box's front is a rendition of a river, a mountain, and sky illuminated in an imitation of stained glass. The bulbs that light the box hum from within.

Avery is transfixed by the light and its glowing colors: the bright blue river, the green mountain, the purple and pink sky. The room smells new to him, too, a thick, floral scent that is coming from the other woman in the room with us—the audiologist, who will retest the hearing in Avery's left ear.

She's a tall, thin woman with short brown hair. She's wearing a lavender twin set that looks soft, like cashmere, and pleated khaki pants. Her clothes are so stylish, and stainable, that I think she must not have kids. We shake hands and I say, "Thank you for meeting us, Doctor." She does not correct me—only later do I learn that she's not a doctor.

We'd arranged this meeting by phone, and her instructions were explicit, if impractical: we were to keep Avery awake all morning, and we were not to feed him. When we got to the hospital, he should be so tired that after one feeding he'd fall into a deep sleep, which is when she'd test him. But Avery's not falling asleep.

"I'll give you ten minutes, and if he's not sleeping, we'll have to go ahead. I have another appointment at three," she tells me, then leaves the room for a moment. I'm out of options. Avery is past the point of sleep—he's overtired. I try to soothe him, try to block out the colors of the light box and the sweet perfume smell by pulling him into me, holding him close. Why we are here, in the chapel instead of an office or an exam room, is unclear. He wiggles and squirms, mesmerized. The woman returns, frowning when she sees Avery is awake.

"We'll do what we can," she says gamely, I think, until she jams a probe into Avery's left ear. The probe is the size of an earplug, pointy on one end and round at the other, connected to a wire that runs to what looks like a laptop. The woman sits on one of the beige stacking chairs, the computer on another, and I am leaning into her, offering Avery up. He's crying so hard that his whole face is red. She's awkward with him and I can tell that the crying is annoying her. What I can't tell is if she's uncomfortable with all babies, or babies with Down syndrome.

"Can you keep him still, please?" she asks me. I try. Avery wails. I hold him tighter. She types something into the laptop. I want to ask her how long this will take, because I can't hold Avery like this for much longer, but she dismisses me with a firm, "Shush."

We do our best, Avery and me. But his wailing turns to hyperventilating, his whole tiny body shaking, and I begin to cry, too. "He was in the NICU for five weeks," I begin, as if reminding her of this fact will change things, but it's over. The big clock at the back of the chapel shows two minutes to three. We've run out of time.

"Look, this isn't working. You'll have to reschedule. Next time make sure he's sleeping. Otherwise, we'll have to put him under." She's cross with us, with me. I'd wanted her to like me— for us to be allies, two players on the same team, team Avery. I'd wanted the hearing test to be successful.

I mumble something about checking our calendar. "I'll get back to you," I say.

"I'd prefer you schedule it now," she answers.

For a moment, I think about the upcoming weeks, trying to imagine when we might come back down. But I'm resistant to the idea. I don't want to deprive Avery of his milk, or his sleep. And I don't want to put him in the hospital again, especially for sedation. It doesn't seem right to me.

"I can't," I say. "I have to check with my husband."

"Well, I suppose that's okay," she says, with a tinge of suspicion. "You'll need to reschedule, though. We'll be calling you," she says, vaguely threatening. Whatever feelings of goodwill I have toward her evaporate. I resent her comments, and her. It was a mistake to bring him here, to hand him over to this woman who jammed a pointy object in his ear and became angry when he cried.

And I hate myself for letting her do it. What kind of a mother am I? I feel like a fool; worse, like a failure. I've let Avery down.

When we get home, I call our family doctor. I explain what happened, and how uneasy I feel about it. I tell him about the withholding food, and about the next test, which will involve sedation.

"I feel uncomfortable with it," I say. "I'm barely used to him being off the monitor. He has reflux troubles. It doesn't feel right to me." I float these thoughts out to our doctor, and even as I'm speaking them aloud, I think, *You sound like an overprotective nut.* I brace myself for my doctor's reaction.

Instead, he surprises me. "Absolutely," he says. "Avery shouldn't be sedated. Don't reschedule the test. We can wait and do an OAE when he's a bit older. I'm going to call the audiologist when I get off the phone with you and tell her that she made a mistake here."

"She's not a doctor?" I ask.

"No. She's a licensed audiologist."

"Thank you. I really appreciate you backing me up on this."

"No problem. I'm glad you called."

I hang up the phone, feeling overwhelmed again. In this instance, I didn't like being right. I'd rather have people in our lives we can trust.

A typical day for us goes something like this: Avery always wakes at five a.m., our little alarm clock. Bennett follows. The house is dark, except for the little light in the kitchen above the stove. Tom makes coffee. In the sleepy half-light, I change Avery's diaper, then change Bennett's diaper. I put them both in the Pack 'n Play. I turn on some music, usually Mozart or sometimes Brahms. The babies are content like this, listening to the music and looking at the changing light, for fifteen minutes or so, and I use the time to get dressed. When they begin to fuss, I turn on the light by the couch, flip the babies onto their tummies, and add some new toys for them to look at, which is good for another fifteen minutes. Tom goes down the hill to the office, or out to a friend's place in the country. He's working on a new book about how to train a colt. Some days, he works with the horse; other days, he writes about it.

I drink my coffee, watching the babies, the sun coming up over the mountains. Soon Carter is awake. I make him a glass of milk with Ovaltine and put a videotape in for him; lately, his favorite is Elmo. While he's watching it, I feed Bennett and put him to sleep in the bouncy seat. Next I feed Avery, and he sleeps in the swing. I set up Carter with a preschool program on the computer, and while he works on it, I empty the dishwasher, load the washing machine, and think about dinner. I rush through these chores because if I can get them all done, I can rest for a minute. It feels as if we've already lived a full day.

By eleven a.m. both babies are up again. This time I feed Avery first, so that I can keep him upright for a half hour before putting him back down on the floor to play with the baby gym. Bennett is next, and while I feed him, I open the door so Carter can play outside on the screened porch. When he returns, we make messes in the kitchen, like baking bread. Carter measures the flour, the yeast, the water, and helps knead the dough. We roll it into logs and make the shapes of the alphabet, *A* for Avery, *B* for Bennett, *C* for Carter.

Afternoons, there are more feedings. Then I take Carter and the babies for a walk in the double stroller. I'm bone-tired by now: I can feel the exhaustion in every part of my body. My mind wanders and I have trouble keeping track of things—once I put the television remote in the fridge; another time I found a sippy cup full of milk in the cupboard. Nothing gets done but watching the clock until six, when Tom returns and we all eat supper. Then baths and bedtime. If everything goes smoothly, the children are asleep by seven. Tom and I stay up another hour together, and then all of us are in bed by eight.

Avery and Carter sleep soundly. Bennett does not. He's up every three hours, sometimes every two. He wakes as if in pain, and I rock him, and hold him, and nurse him, until I can't do it anymore, and then I hand him off to Tom. I don't know how much longer we can keep this up—Bennett, Tom, and me with jangled nerves and broken sleep.

After a particularly bad night, I tell Tom that I'm going to take Bennett to see our doctor again. Something isn't right. A baby shouldn't cry so much. I call the office, and although there are no appointments available, the nurse I speak with says to come in anyway, and the doc will see us in between his other patients.

Tom stays home with Avery and Carter, and I drive Bennett to town. The nurse has me undress him and we wait in a supply room, which is the only available space. Bennett's little body is shivering and I hold him close to me, wrapped in the knit baby blanket Joyce gave us. I rock him next to my body, I whisper to him, I kiss the top of his head, all the while thinking, *Please, let everything be okay.*

Our doctor appears, unwraps Bennett, and looks him over, then says, "I'm going to send you to Missoula. I want you to see the pediatric surgeon there. I'll try and get you an appointment today." He looks concerned and I take my cues from him; if he thinks it's serious, then I do, too.

His nurse comes into the supply room with a slip of paper. We have an appointment in the afternoon and I don't even have time to go home if I want to make it to Missoula. I ask to use the phone and call Tom to tell him the plan. He's worried now, too, and has many questions, but I have no answers. I tell him that I'll call him when I know more.

Bennett sleeps most of the way down to the hospital. He wakes in time for the walk through the building to the office, and his howls echo along the corridors. The nurses hear us and come out into the hall to meet me. I hand one our insurance cards, and tell her about Bennett: seven weeks premature, fraternal twin, feeding issues, maybe colic. The other guides us to an exam room and tells me the doctor will come right away. She does: she's a middle-aged woman with short black hair and is wearing a maroon sweater, a flowered skirt, and a string of pearls.

"I'm Dr. Manktelow, but you can call me Dr. Anne. Everybody does. It's easier to say," she says with a British accent.

Dr. Anne examines Bennett quickly, settling on his belly button, which pooches out like a small thumb. "Has it always been like this?" she asks.

"Yes, I think so," I say. "It's always stuck out. I can't say if it's gotten worse, though."

"What this is called is an umbilical hernia," she begins. "The muscles of the stomach are one of the last things to fuse together before birth. We often see this in premature babies, that the muscles haven't closed properly. In Bennett's case, part of his intestine has pushed out through the opening."

She explains it all so clearly, and it makes such good sense as told by her in her lovely accent, that I feel immediately relieved. Here's an answer to all of Bennett's crying. I expect her to tell me that we should wait for him to outgrow it, and send us on our way. Instead, I hear her say something about options, and techniques for repair.

I interrupt. "Um, excuse me. What are we talking about?"

"I think this needs to be repaired. In surgery. It would require general anesthesia, and an overnight stay in the PICU. But I think it's severe enough to warrant the procedure."

"I was hoping you'd tell me he'd outgrow it," I begin.

"That's one option, but . . ."

I sigh.

"What is it?" she asks.

"There is always a 'but' these days," I say.

She smiles at me with empathy. "I'd like to call a colleague of mine to discuss it. Afterward, I'll be in touch. The best thing for you to do is to go home and I'll call you there."

I dial the number of Dr. Anne's office, then hang up. Dial it, hang up. It will be nothing, I tell myself. But I have a sick feeling in the pit of my stomach. Time passes so slowly. Tom has stayed home and I do nothing but hold Bennett, who nurses and nurses. I wrap us both in a fuzzy blanket and sit and watch the light move across the lake. Morning, midmorning, midday. Late afternoon, dusk, sunset, dark. I can't get anything done.

Early the next morning Dr. Anne's nurse calls. Yes, surgery is recommended. We will have to be at Community Medical Center by 10:00 a.m. Friday. I'm not supposed to feed anything to Bennett from 5:30 a.m. on. He can have breast milk until 7:30 a.m., then nothing else. "Will this be okay?" the nurse asks.

"Yes," I say. "Yes, it will be fine. It will all be fine."

I tell Tom. He's supposed to be gone this weekend. I don't want him to postpone his trip; I don't want the surgery to wait. I can't make any decisions. I'm having trouble thinking clear thoughts. All I want to do is hold Bennett and rock back and forth, back and forth in the rocking chair.

"I'm sorry," I say.

"I'm sorry, too," Tom says.

"No, I'm sorry for all of it. I'm sorry I wanted more kids. I'm sorry I put us through this. I had no idea. I had no idea it could get this bad," I say, crying and rocking. "About Avery, too—it's my fault. I did this to us. It's me. It's my fault."

"Jen, don't," he says.

"I'll make this right, I promise you," I say. "You'll see. I'll make it right."

"Jen, stop. It's not your fault. There's nothing to make right. It's all going to be okay. Sometimes hard things happen to people. It's no one's fault. It's life."

"But if we had stopped with Carter, if we—"

"But we didn't. We have three beautiful boys. It's all going to be okay. It will. Get some rest. You need sleep. We'll make it through this, you'll see. You'll feel better after you get some rest."

"It was my old eggs that did this."

"You can't say that. It could have been me. We don't know what caused it. We'll never know. And it doesn't matter. What we have now is what matters. Life is hard, but it's good, too. Hard, but good. Don't forget that." He kisses me on the top of the head. "Try to sleep."


I don't remember falling asleep, but when I wake, Bennett is in my arms and we're still in the rocker. The sky is gray and the light outside is faint. Late afternoon. I feel better for all the crying, and for Tom's words. I don't believe for one minute that it isn't my fault, but I appreciate that he cares enough about me to protect me, even from myself.

I wander out into the family room, Bennett still in my arms, and everything's been arranged while I slept—Tom canceled his trip; he'll stay home to take care of Avery and Carter. And I'm to take Bennett back down to Missoula for the surgery, another drive to the hospital in the dark early morning.

Bennett is in his coming-home outfit, the one that was much too big on him when we left the NICU. Now it's almost too small. His little white hat is perched on his head at a jolly angle. It makes me smile, and cry. It's all so much harder, now that we've had time to know him, to love him.

I leave breast milk for Avery in the fridge in the little plastic Baggies. I take the big blue breast pump. I pack my fleece socks, and a photo of the babies from the NICU, and a photo of Tom with Carter on his shoulders, all good-luck charms that I think might somehow keep us safe, but it doesn't feel like enough. I dig out the *woo-woo cards* from my stay in the hospital, which I'd tucked in my journal. I place the cards on either side of the two photos, and layer one in between, so that we are protected on all sides.

I drive through the darkness past the places of our lives: Lori's house, where Carter sometimes plays in the summers, Gina's house, Sarah's house. The little restaurant across from the fire hall where we took Tom's parents to dinner to celebrate our pregnancy. And the fire hall itself, where the firemen pooled their money to buy us hundreds of Huggies Supremes. Claudia's house, then Etta's, around the bend in the road, past the greenhouse owned by a woman who sells me flowers in the spring. It's my little neck of the woods. Moving through it, from one safe place to another, gives me courage.

The highway is a ribbon of asphalt through the middle of the still-sleepy valley. The sun is rising over the mountains and I can feel it warm the left side of my face. Everything seems full of portent, even the way the sunlight breaks over the mountains, but what it signifies, I don't yet know.

We pass by the familiar little roads—Beaverhead, Duck, Kicking Horse—and the farmsteads and the houses. Eagle Pass, Gunlock, Post Creek, and the green highway sign, MISSOULA— 40 MI. Before long, the road widens to four lanes and we are in Busytown, with its stoplights and fast-food restaurants and box stores. Traffic. People on their way to work. Bennett is awake and fussing. I see the blue hospital sign and follow the road past the Holiday Gas Station, past the Village Health Care Senior Residence, past the green grass of the golf course. The sprinklers are just coming on, as if announcing our arrival. The sign at Community Medical Center reads, 1565 BABIES A YEAR . . . AND COUNTING!

We are here.

A nurse tells me that Dr. Anne will be right with us and she gives me a clipboard, with a form for me to sign.

"It's standard," she explains. "But you should read it."

It says that as Bennett's guardian, I understand that complications can occur as a result of general anesthesia that can cause death. By signing the form, I understand and accept this risk. My hand is shaking and I have to steady it to write my name.


We wait in the room next to surgery. There's an older couple sitting near the lamp, each reading a magazine. I wonder which one of them is sick. There's a young woman near the nurse's desk. She, too, has a baby in a baby carrier. I take Bennett out of his car seat and hold him.

The nurse calls Bennett's name. She tells me I have to say my good-byes in the waiting room. My eyes well up with tears. I can't do it. I can't let my baby go. The young mother looks away, the older woman smiles at me. I turn my back to all of them, and hold Bennett tighter, facing the wall.

I hear Dr. Anne's voice behind me. "Is there a problem?" she asks.

"I'm having a little trouble," I say.

"It's hard, when they're so small," she says. "Why don't we let you come as far as recovery?" I turn to her. She's dressed in pale green scrubs, still wearing her string of pearls. Her arms are outstretched, waiting for Bennett. She takes him, but I'm allowed to hold his hand.

We walk through the swinging double doors. The nurse separates us, Bennett going with Dr. Anne. His little white hat drops to the floor. I pick it up. The nurse sits me in a chair and tells me to wait, it should be about an hour.

"Would you like anything?" she asks.

"Some water, please," I manage.

I have my bag with me, and Bennett's bag, and his little hat that fell off when they took him. I lay it on my lap and smooth it. The nurse brings me a sip of water in a paper cup. I drink the water and crumple the cup into a ball. I look around for a wastebasket, but can't find one. I don't know what to do with the crumpled cup—it seems like too big of a decision to make right now. I put it in my pocket.

My hand returns to the hat on my lap. I finger the loose thread on the teddy bear. I check the clock. Time is passing. I bring the hat to my face and inhale. It smells like babies, and like home. I think of Tom and Carter and Avery. I imagine what they are doing. Probably eating lunch, almost ready for nap time. I put the hat back down in my lap and straighten it out again.

I hear hospital sounds, the clinking of the pipes and the hum of the HVAC. I think what a fuzzy place this is. Time stops here. It's as if I never left. I'm in the same recovery bay I was in all those months ago, when my nose was so red and I couldn't stop scratching it. I can feel the itch, even now.

And yet it's been a lifetime. Two lifetimes.

I sit, suspended in the moment, not moving forward, not moving back. I haven't thought of Sandy B. since I was pregnant, but she comes into my mind. I think of her hug to me, a gift. I wish I had that hug again, and the feeling of well-being it brought. Remembering her brings fresh tears, for Avery. Avery is so soft. His lip quivers when he cries; he sucks his hand to soothe himself.

I wish he were here for me to hold. I miss him. I want both my babies, just as they are, and I want to be with them for a long, long time. I lift Bennett's little white hat to my face to dry my eyes and I think again of life's sandpaper. I wonder, how much more wearing down do I need, and how much more can I take?

Watching them wheel Bennett back to me on a silver gurney, his little body naked except for a diaper and a patch of gauze over his belly button, his eyes groggy but open, and the nurse's, "He did great, Mom," I feel gratitude pulse through me like blood, flowing into every cell of my body. All that matters to me is that we are here, healthy and full of life. And we have each other. I can see that, now. It's taken me a long time, but finally, I can see.

# 8

### ❧

# I Think I Remember

There was a time before Avery, a time that to me now, looking back, seems silver and smooth and shiny, like the face of a
new quarter. Then the twins are born, and life is tossed in the air,
flipped high in the blue sky, spinning end over end. And when it
lands, instead of heads, we are tails. It's still the same shiny coin,
it's still smooth and silver. And yet, everything is completely different.

The territory is familiar enough that sometimes I forget it's
new, until something happens that reminds me my life is changed,
and I have that flipping sensation again, my mind spinning as I try
to regain my balance. Something as simple as a message on the answering machine. Sarah's voice, saying, "The Blue Mountain All
Women's Run is this weekend. A bunch of us will be going down
and you could come for the ride, if you want. Let me know?"

The Blue Mountain All Women's Run is an annual event
sponsored each October by the Blue Mountain Clinic, a medical
center in Missoula that combines traditional and alternative therapies. One of the services the clinic provides is abortion. I've never
been there. I haven't participated in the run. Each year, I plan to
go, but something always comes up.

Though I missed out in the past, I've heard about the day.
There is excitement (sometimes a crowd protests outside the
clinic), there is camaraderie (women of many ages coming to-

gether for a shared cause), and there's fun: women saying good-bye to their husbands and children for a day of carpooling in the family Subaru or minivan, but instead of driving to kindergarten or soccer, it's a carpool of grown-ups going on an adventure. After the event, everyone goes to lunch at the Mustard Seed.

I used to want to be a part of it. But this year, I don't know that I'd go even if I could. The reason for my change of heart is a statistic: 92 percent of women who receive a prenatal diagnosis of Down syndrome terminate the pregnancy.

Before Avery, I would have said, *Fine. That's their choice*. And I would have meant it. Now, on this new flipped-coin landscape, I can't say that anymore. I take the termination statistic personally. Nine out of ten women at the Blue Mountain All Women's Run would make a different choice about Avery. He's the child they would not have had.

I don't blame them for not wanting my life. I don't know how to make sense of it myself most days. But then I think of Avery. Sucking his thumb, his foot. His big blue eyes, watching me. I feel the weight of what the statistic means: it's exactly ten pounds nine ounces, the most recent weight of Avery.

Sometimes in the night, I wake with a start, believing I've heard the alarm on his monitor. It's quiet, so I search for the glowing green-green-green blink of its lights. I don't see that either, and I'm filled with a dreadful panic. Where is Avery, where is my Avery?

And then I remember.

In the beginning, I couldn't imagine a life with him. I'd wake from dreams in which Carter was my only child, and the realities of my second pregnancy would darken my consciousness like spilled ink.

Now I can't stand the thought of life without him. I go to him, after my nightmares, and gently touch my hand to his chest, letting the steady rhythm of his heart slow the beating of my own.

Tom is home and gone, home and gone for work, traveling to the little communities and bookstores across Montana to talk about writing. He's the shy type, preferring to put his thoughts on paper rather than speak them aloud, so for him, book promotion requires a great effort. But he comes home happy, so he must be getting something good out of these trips—perspective, maybe, or appreciation, or even admiration. I don't think either one of us can get enough support and I want him to take it all in. Welcome every kindness.

We've arranged to have help each time Tom is away. Tom's parents came first. Then friends filled in. Now my dad is flying out from Chicago to meet the babies. He's coming without his wife, Pam, who can't make it.

I'm hoping to have a serious conversation with him. I want to ask him about life—mine, his, and mostly, Avery's. I want his opinion because he was raised in a family with three children; Tom and I now have three children. And my dad's older brother was born with physical challenges and other issues, things I know little of because it's not usually discussed.

If I could, I'd have this conversation with my grandmother. I'd ask her how to do this—how do you raise a family of three children, one with special needs? My grandmother is gone, though, and my dad is the only one I can ask, but I don't know how. Ours is a relationship of deeds, not words.

During my first semester in college, I flew home for my grandmother's funeral. There was so much to talk about, then—my mediocre grades, my broken budget, my lack of direction. His life, too, and the growing realization that he and my mom would soon divorce. And our mutual loss of Gram, a woman we both loved deeply. If ever there was a time for talk it was then, but we didn't speak about any of it. Instead, the last morning of my visit, I woke in my childhood bed, surrounded by white and gold little-girl furniture, pink and red bows on the bedside lamp. Outside the bedroom door were my black shoes, neatly placed side by side and gleaming with new polish, ready for my journey back to school. My dad had shined them in the night, while I was sleeping.

Or a more recent memory: the day of my marriage to Tom. It had been a stressful week of a thousand details, a hundred minor things gone wrong and corrected, all settling in to the final moment, when I was supposed to walk down the grass to Tom, who was waiting for me at the waterfront with the minister, the groomsmen, and the bridesmaids. I knew I wanted to make this commitment, recognized it as good and right, yet I was unable to move. I was shaking so hard I couldn't walk. I tried to speak, but nothing came out. My dad took my arm, wrapped it over his, patted my hand, and led the way. All I had to do was hold on.

These are the moments of my life with my dad. In all our time together, I have never asked the questions I most need answers to. And now, I'm hoping it isn't too late.

When he arrives, I see him as if for the first time, noticing how much he looks like Avery, Avery and me, me and Gram. All of us, branches on a family tree. If there is a gene for snoring, we share it. Thick hair, all of us. Tall. My dad is six feet four, and has dark brown hair and a mustache. When *Magnum, P.I.* was a popular show, people would say he looked like Tom Selleck.

Carter has come out of the house with me. Bennett is inside, sleeping, and I have Avery in my arms. Carter eyes his grandpa from behind my leg. "Say hi to Grandpa," I tell him. "Give him a hug."

Carter goes to my dad and hugs him seriously, carefully. It has been a year since they last saw each other.

I hug him, too. "Good to see you," I say. "Thanks for coming." I have that familiar feeling of happiness and nervousness that I've always felt around him. A feeling of being awkward and comfortable at the same time. I'm ten years old again, watching my dad cook steaks on the grill, hoping he notices me sitting beside him, waiting for him to let me hold the barbecue tongs or refill his drink or run into the house and tell Mom that dinner is almost ready.

Dad says, "And this must be Avery." I think he might ask to hold Avery, but he doesn't. His arms are full of luggage.

"Let's go in," I say.

We walk single file, my dad, then Carter, then me with Avery, his blue eyes shining, his tongue flicking in and out, tasting the air. Part of me wants to blurt out my questions, or say something like, "We need to talk!" so that there will be no going back. Another part of me resists. I hesitate and the moment passes silently, quietly, unnoticed by anyone but me.

After Dad unpacks, we begin dinner. Each time he visits, he cooks steaks, thick slabs of marbled red meat that are ordinarily too expensive for us, cuts like rib eyes or T-bones. The wind off the lake is coming down from the north, Canadian air, and the sunlight is weak and thin, but we don't change our plans because of the cold—we don't even consider it.

Since childhood, I've watched my dad prepare and cook meat. It always begins with a clean cookie sheet. The steaks, freed from their foam and cellophane, are rinsed in the sink and patted dry with a paper towel. The meat is placed on the tray, sprinkled with garlic salt, then pepper. Mustard powder. Worcestershire sauce. Olive oil. Rub it into a paste. Turn the steaks over and repeat.

My dad is showing Carter this process. I'm dangling a multicolored Whoozit over the Pack 'n Play, temporarily distracting the babies. I can hear Dad telling Carter something about "when your mother was your age," and I feel like an eavesdropper. It's odd to hear my dad referring to me as someone's mother. With him, I still think of myself as a child. I have that flipping sensation again, of my life turning on end and landing upside down, or inside out.

Dad and Carter take the tray of meat out to the porch. Carter comes inside and asks me to get Grandpa a glass of wine, only instead of waiting for it and bringing it back out, as I would have done when I was his age, he goes into his bedroom and begins playing with his LEGOS. I open the bottle Dad has brought, a red zinfandel from Spain, and pour a bit into a short, squat juice glass—both my dad and Tom think long-stemmed wineglasses are fussy and pretentious. I bring the drink outside.

"Here you go, Dad." I place the glass on the porch railing. It's cold, but the lake is deep blue and the mountains are rich with the colors of fall—yellows and oranges and shocking lime green, bright white snow on the highest peaks.

I think about saying, *Dad, what was it like for you, growing up?* or *Dad, what advice do you have for me?* but I don't. The words will simply not come out.

"Can I get you anything else? Do you want your coat?" I ask instead.

"Thanks, no," he says. "I'm fine."

If I were still a child, I would stay outside with him and watch the rows of tiny whitecaps form and disappear on the lake. Or I'd look at the sky changing from blue to pink to purple to black. Or I'd sit and listen to the sizzle of the steaks and wait for the occasional flare-up, exciting when seen from a safe distance, my dad by my side. I wish I could go back. There were no questions that were too big, and my dad knew the answer to everything.

I'm mother to children of my own now, and I feel the tug of them pulling me back inside the house. It's a real pull; it's also my excuse.

"I better get back to the babies," I say. "Holler if you need anything."

Dad has a new cell phone that looks like two credit cards hinged together. It rings off and on throughout dinner, playing a little melody, part of a song. Mostly, it's Pam calling. She wants to know what we're doing. Dad hands the phone to me to say hello.

I take it gingerly, dubiously, doubtfully. Growing up, I was never allowed to talk on the phone at dinner. Tom and I let the machine get any calls that come while we're eating. Taking this tiny phone makes me uncomfortable.

"Hello?" I say. I can hear Pam's voice, but it sounds far away. She's asking how we are.

"Everything's great!" I say. It's difficult to hear over the static, and some of what I'm listening to makes no sense. Words are missing.

I try to speak louder, and I repeat myself. "Everything is great! Everything is great!" I yell and repeat, yell and repeat, over and over, like shouting a mantra.

The yelling is too much. Avery, who's been sitting in his high chair sucking on his fist, begins to cry. Bennett, also in his high chair, starts fussing because Avery is upset. The once-quiet house is a cacophony.

I give up and hand the phone back to Dad, who steps out on the porch, hoping for better reception. I look at the clock. Two more hours. In that time, I have to give the babies baths and fresh diapers, and get them in their sleepers. I have to wash Carter's face, help him brush his teeth, and change his clothes, too. I shovel some food into Carter's mouth, and go to Avery. I unfasten the clips on the high chair's safety harness and hold him under one arm. Using my other hand, I unclip Bennett from his high chair, and roll him onto my hip. I'm already so tired.

Out the big picture window, I can see Dad sitting on the porch, talking on the phone. He's not yelling, or struggling, so the reception must be okay. He's sitting with his back to the house, looking out. I try to see what he sees. The light is settling over the tree-covered slopes. Everything is pink, then purple with night.

I can see my reflection in the window glass, too, a baby under each arm, pushing Carter forward through the kitchen, pointing the way to the bath with my leg, so much hanging on me, hanging on to me. My parents were divorced more than twenty years ago; since then, our distance has become a habit. We are so loosely connected—my mother, my father, my sister, and I. A single silver thread holds us together, the thread of memory.

A brother, gone thirty years. A mother, gone twenty. Dad, sitting in the cedar chair on the porch. I see him, and I see us in him. I don't want to push, don't want to ask for too much, because I can't bear to lose what little we have. The thought of it makes me feel vulnerable, and I'm sick of feeling vulnerable.

I shepherd my little herd into the bathroom, twist the knobs on the water in the tub, and strip clothes from little bodies. The water fills. I add a plastic boat, a toy frog. Carter gets in the tub. I spread two clean towels on the floor and place Bennett on one, Avery on the other. They will get a wipe down with baby wash and warm water from the tub. My three boys. And I am the mother.

"I love you, Carter. You know that, right?" I say.

"Yes, Mommy, I know. I love you, too."

"Thank you, honey. You know that if you ever wanted to ask me something, you could, right?" I say.

"Yes, I know," he says. He pauses for a moment, thinking, then asks, "You know frogs, Mommy?"

"Yes."

"Where do they sleep?"

"On a moss bed with a leaf blanket and the moon for a nightlight," I say.

"Inside or outside the pond?"

"Umm, outside, I think."

"I get it," he says, satisfied. "So the fish don't eat them."


Instead of telling old family stories, my dad gives me something new. Forty-five minutes from our home is a warehouse store that's part of a national chain. The store requires shoppers to purchase a membership, something Tom and I have never done, but Dad and Pam have been members for years. Dad wants to take me there.

We plan the trip with military precision. I pack provisions for Carter—extra sippies, cheese crackers, and M&Ms in case of an emergency. For the babies, I bring spare outfits, the diaper bag, wipes, extra bottles, blankets, coats and hats. Toys, too: rattles, Taggies, a soft-padded mirror, and the Whoozit. I check the car—gas, tires, oil—everything is a go. We bring the babies out first, get their carriers settled, then strap Carter in his car seat, three in a row across the back. Dad rides in the passenger seat and I drive. Before we've even reached the mailbox, Carter and the babies are asleep. Soon enough, we reach the big gray building I've passed by many times before but never entered. Here I turn in, and park.

The first thing I notice about warehouse shopping are the giant carts, with two spaces for children in the front and an extra-wide basket in the back. I strap Bennett into the BabyBjörn, because I think it'll work the best, and I leave Avery in his car seat and put him in the shopping cart. Dad pushes it to the store. Carter, Bennett, and I trail close behind.

At the entrance, an employee checks Dad's membership card and we're waved into the massive space. It's the largest building Carter has ever been in and he grips my hand a little tighter. We follow Dad as he pushes Avery and the shopping cart around the store, slowly filling it with diapers and wipes, bananas, steak. Jelly beans for Carter. Coffee for me and Tom. As we're shopping, Dad tells me about the things he and Pam buy—wine, cheese, coconut-crusted shrimp—so different from the supplies today, paper towels and Simple Green and Febreze. At each aisle's end, there are little cups of samples, like chicken noodle soup or wild salmon burgers or a fizzy energy drink. It occurs to me that I haven't been out of the house in a long while. It feels like a party.

I haven't gone out for several reasons. First, there are the logistics—it takes a lot of effort to get three children anywhere. Second, since the NICU, I've turned into a germaphobe. Nothing seems safe or sanitary enough, not even our home, which I accept by telling myself that our germs are familiar germs. And finally, I'm not sure what to expect.

I'm overly aware of Avery, constantly checking on him and trying to gauge other people's reactions to him. I think things like *That lady gave me a knowing smile.* Or, *There's no way that couple guessed anything—they just thought he was cute.* Or, *For heaven's sake, Avery, keep your tongue in your mouth!*

I'm having all these internal stirrings, wondering and worrying what people are thinking of us, but Dad doesn't seem bothered at all. He pushes Avery and smiles proudly at the other shoppers. I take my cue from him, and do the same.

If my dad is about not talking, my mom is the opposite. With her, ideas are meant to be turned over and discussed. It's her way of understanding the world, by wrapping words around it. She visits from Chicago shortly after Dad leaves. Having her here so soon after my dad brings back memories of their relationship. Mom is a Democrat and Dad is a Republican, and much of their marital discord found its way into politics. Mine was a childhood of power struggles couched in policy.

"Republicans are selfish and only think of themselves," my mother would argue.

"Democrats spend too much. They won't accept fiscal responsibility," my dad would counter.

"It's exactly like a Republican to turn his back on the women and children. Where are they when you need them?" Mom would say.

"Democrats let their emotions get the best of them," Dad would answer.

As a result, I've been unable to commit to any political party. If I side with the Democrats, I feel as if I am abandoning my dad.

If I choose Republicans, I'm rejecting my mom. And if I chose neither, I let them both down. For me, it's a familiar quandary.

I have another childhood memory, of my mother in a chartreuse dress, her feathered hair sprayed into waves that peeked out from either side of her Brownie camera, like wings. "Say limburger." My mom, always taking photos, posing us, arranging our lives into the perfect picture. It made me feel as if someone were watching, someone who needed to be impressed. The film landed in shoe boxes under her bed, where they accumulated, hundreds of little black rolls all waiting to be developed.

The mother wearing the chartreuse dress was young. We'd recently moved from the Midwest to a new subdivision in northern California. I think it was the first time she really felt alone, away from her family, away from her mother. She'd meet up with the other neighborhood moms in the afternoons and they'd walk around and around the block, pushing strollers, holding little hands grimy with peanut butter and apple juice, to pass the time.

It was the height of the seventies and Mom played us a Marlo Thomas record called *Free to Be . . . You and Me*, with songs about equal rights in which mommies have families and careers both. My mom, my sister, and I would drive around in her white Ford Granada, singing along to the AM radio. Mom encouraged us to believe the world would be welcoming to us, more so than it had been to her, and her mother before her. She wanted us to be ready, to grow into strong women, her two budding feminists.

Sometimes I'd sit on the edge of the bed and watch her get dressed. She had long red fingernails and wore matching red lipstick. I remember the smell of her, a combination of hairspray and perfume, which she kept on a little mirrored tray on her dresser. She'd let me twist open the lids and smell the fragrances—White Shoulders, Chanel No. 5, Opium—then she'd reach down and dab a bit of whatever she was wearing on each of my wrists.

On the weekends, my parents had parties. I recall tables on

the patio lit with candles, casting long shadows across the swimming pool and into the persimmon trees. The women wore cocktail dresses and high heels, laughing and talking. The clink of ice in glasses, the tapping of heels across cement. Mom was calling for my sister and me to come out and say good night. I felt awkward and shy in the spotlight and had none of my mother's ability to rise to the occasion, as she called it.

We were out on the patio when I saw the flames. A candle had set a basket of napkins on fire. I stood terrified and mesmerized. My mother paused midsentence, saw what I saw, walked to the table, picked up the flaming basket, and tossed it into the pool. The guests laughed and cheered. Hooray! She did this all without interrupting her conversation. My mother was like that. She could take the oxygen right out of a room, leaving everyone breathless. She was a force as bright as the sun, and I was in her orbit.


It's from my mother that I learned what it is to be a woman: an awesome honor and responsibility both. When she visits from Chicago, I expect that she'll want to discuss Avery, which I'm not ready to do. But I'm wrong. Mom is more quiet than I've ever known her to be. She's holding herself back, giving me my space, trying to let me find my own words without inserting hers. I keep thinking she'll bring it up, and I prepare myself to dodge the subject, which makes me defensive and always on guard. This in itself would be cause enough for discussion; it's a vicious cycle, one I can't seem to get out of, but Mom lets it go.

Instead of talking, she works. She feeds Avery gently and carefully so he won't spit up. She empties the dishwasher and sweeps the floor. She cooks dinner for Tom and me, things she thinks Tom will like, such as spaghetti with meat sauce, and she wraps everything in saran wrap labeled with a black Sharpie, *Turkey sandwich with lettuce, tomato, mayonnaise and mustard.*

*Pickle on the side.* She plays with Carter, building endless LEGO creations. And when she speaks of Avery, everything she says is positive: "His skin is translucent," or "He's beautiful," or "He's a dear. He's a love." She says, "One thing about children with Down syndrome—they seem to bring out the good in people."

Mom takes lots of photographs, too, using a disposable panoramic camera, which she likes for its wide, long pictures. She doesn't try to pose us like I remember from my childhood—instead, she takes what she calls candids. When she gets back to Chicago, she has the film developed and sends us duplicates. A wide-angled shot of our little lawn that makes it look huge, lush and green. A panoramic photo of the mountains that seems as if the view goes on forever. Carter, sideways, with impossibly long legs. Me and Carter and the babies—I look very tired, but we seem happy.

The last photo is a picture of Avery in panorama, alone. He is glassy-eyed, spacey. The bridge of his nose is flat and wide. His tongue is sticking out. He looks bad. He looks retarded. I rip the photo into tiny pieces and stick it in the trash, beneath the coffee grounds and the empty milk carton, where no one can see.

I still watch too much television. The Tour de France is over, but I've switched to talk shows. I can't watch the actual news, as it makes me feel helpless and weepy, but the distilled version surrounded by fashion advice and cooking tips helps me pass the time.

In the mornings, I watch NBC's *Today.* I tell myself that I tune in to get information about the weather, but since I rarely go outside, I'm not fooling anyone, not even myself. Katie, Matt, Al, and Ann are my current support van; they help me keep my mind occupied as I move through the day—the never-ending loop around the oversize chair, from Boppy to Pack 'n Play to

Exersaucer to Gymini to baby swing; the dozen feedings and changings, two nap times and a bath time that comprise my current life.

One morning, as I'm taking Bennett from his tummy time at the Gymini to the Boppy, so that Avery can have his tummy time, I hear Ann Curry's voice announcing new research that suggests women will soon be able to harvest and freeze eggs for IVF at a later date, with an encouraging success rate. Ann is cheerful, and says that the findings will give women the same kinds of reproductive choices men have. By freezing their eggs, she says, women can circumvent the biological clock and delay pregnancy indefinitely.

Her message has an unspoken subtext, which I hear loud and clear: the likelihood of having a baby with Down syndrome increases after the age of thirty-five. By freezing "young" eggs, this risk can be reduced. It's as if a friend of mine just called to tell me that I should be happy for her, because she won't ever have to have a child like mine. I don't feel happy. I feel assaulted. I can't get to the television fast enough to turn it off.

Instead of watching television, I read everything I can find that's written by a parent of a child with Down syndrome, such authors as Marilyn Trainer, Barbara Gill, Michael Bérubé, Martha Beck, Vicki Noble, and Pam Vredevelt. These people become my revised and improved support team and each of them offers me something worthwhile: Marilyn Trainer is the mom-next-door with solid, practical advice. Barbara Gill is the wise, gentle friend you'd discuss life with over a cup of herbal tea. Michael Bérubé is the college professor who speaks about the development of intelligence and IQ testing in ways I can understand. Martha Beck is Bérubé's female counterpart, but she also talks about a spiritual side to her experience that I've felt, in my own way, too. Reading about her thoughts makes me feel less shy about my own; my wacky *woo-woo cards* and Sandy B.'s hug, which I've come to think of as the *meaningful hug*. Vicki Noble and Pam Vredevelt talk almost exclusively about faith, and I need them, too—I think of them as points on a spectrum; Vredevelt is the far right of traditional Christianity, and Noble is the far left of alternative spirituality. What I'm learning is simple, and obvious, but is still news to me: there's no one right way to raise a child with Down syndrome. Just as each child is unique, so is each parent. We're all doing the best we can.

The restaurant on the highway near the long road that leads out to our house is no more than a fishing shack, where summer tourists buy six-packs of Budweiser or foam containers of red worms or the requisite permits and licenses. To the side are a few tables, where people can sit and eat plates of fried whitefish or hamburgers with a soda or a beer or one of two kinds of wine—red or white—both from a box. We came here to tell Tom's folks we were pregnant; today we're back, for the first time as a family, to celebrate Tom's birthday. We have the place to ourselves because it's only five o'clock.

The waitress, who also doubles as the bartender and the bait salesperson, helps us settle in to our table. Carter sits next to me, and Tom and I each hold a baby. "Twins?" she asks. I nod.

"They're adorable," she says. I've become an expert on nuances regarding Avery, and I detect nothing but goodwill.

"And you must be the big brother," she says to Carter, who nods his head solemnly. I squeeze Carter's hand and smile at him.

We place our order, and when the food arrives, the waitress offers to take a baby so that one of us can eat. For a minute, I consider it. Avery is easier, which is both a reason to keep him and a reason to share him. While I hesitate, Tom says, "Thanks, but we've got it. We're good."

Bennett grabs at my plate, so I let him hold a French fry. He mashes it into his mouth and begins gumming it while I cut Carter's hamburger into four pieces, a habit so ingrained that I sometimes catch myself cutting my own food into bits, without even thinking about it. Avery sees that Bennett has a fry and reaches for one, too—Tom looks at me to see if it's okay and I shrug. I've become lax compared to how I was with Carter. What's the harm in one French fry?

When we've finished eating, I reach into the side pocket of the diaper bag and pull out a birthday card for Tom. It says all the things I mean to say every day but don't—what a good friend he is to me, what a good father, what a good man. I mean it, every word of it, more than I ever have before.

Inside the card is a crayon drawing of our house, smoke curling out of the chimney, from Carter. He's also drawn us all together, holding hands in a line, biggest to smallest, including two tiny figures each the same size, the babies.

"It's our family," Carter explains, as Tom unfolds the paper.

"What a beautiful job you did," Tom says. I can tell he's touched. It's the best picture Carter has made.

"I didn't help him," I add. "He did it all by himself."

"Happy Birthday, Daddy. I love you," Carter says.

It's a simple night. And yet Tom doesn't seem to mind. Perhaps, like me, he's finding himself thankful for even the smallest of gifts. Cheeseburgers and sodas, a Hallmark card and a homemade picture of our life in crayon: a man and a woman, standing together. A beautiful boy. Two little babies. A warm house full of love, its roof a solid triangle above, pointing to the sky.

# 9

≼⁓

# Some Days Are Better Than Others

Here we are, a family of five sitting in the waiting room of the county health department. It's time to begin immunizations for the babies. There are forms to fill out—name, address, date of birth. Immediately, I stumble. *Do I use their actual date of birth or their adjusted-age date of birth? Or is it my age they want? Why would they want that?*

I go to the woman at the makeshift front desk, really just a corner carved out of the room itself—high white ceilings, two plain couches, industrial carpeting on the floor. A small pile of toys in a corner; *Family Circle* and *People* and *Newsweek* on an end table. A shelf behind the front desk holds school photos of children and a baby bottle filled with Lucite. Inside the bottle, encased in the plastic, are cigarette butts, capsules, and pills—a visual reminder that what you do goes right to your baby. The woman behind the desk has short brown hair, a brown sweater, and a warm smile. She reminds me of cinnamon.

I ask her about the forms and she tells me, in the nicest possible way, to use the date the babies were delivered. She smiles at me, at Tom, at Avery. I return to my seat on the couch and continue. Allergies? *Don't know.* Chicken pox? *Don't think so.* HIV/AIDS? *Probably no; I think I'd remember if there were any blood transfusions, but I can't be sure.* The forms remind me how little I know about my babies; what a poor guardian I've been. I rush through the rest of the questions, answering as best I can, and then I realize something is missing. There isn't a place to put Down syndrome. It doesn't fit anywhere. I add it under "Other." I guess that's what it is: something Other. I put a star by it, then add one more, like the stars in Avery's eyes.

I return the paperwork to the woman behind the desk, and also give her copies of the NICU release papers, the birth certificates, and the well-check forms from our family practitioner. She smiles again and says, "It'll just be a minute."

The children and Tom and I play train—Daddy and Avery are the engine, Carter is a boxcar, Bennett and I are the caboose. While we're shuffling around the floor, the woman organizes our paperwork; then she fills out new medical record cards for us. She has pretty handwriting and the cards are clean and tidy; she slips them into clear plastic protectors for safekeeping.

Our names are called by a nurse with sad eyes and a weary way about her—gentle, quiet, and soft-spoken, she reminds me of our last nurse in the NICU, the one who helped with the babies' releases. She asks who'll get the first shot and Tom and I discuss it: Bennett will cry, certainly; Avery will cry if Bennett is crying. We decide to have Avery go first.

The nurse plunges the needle into Avery's left thigh. His face folds and he crumples into a whole-body frown, which dissolves into a single loud wail. Memories of the NICU come flooding back to me: the powerlessness, the fear, the pain. All the pain. Avery is crying; Bennett joins him; Carter looks as if he'll cry, too. Tears well up in my eyes. I reach for Avery and hold him; I'm already holding Bennett. There's not enough room for the nurse to give Bennett his shot, but I'm not willing to let go.

Tom removes Avery from my arms and whispers, "It'll be okay." I hold Bennett for his shot. Again, the needle, the memories. And then it's over and we're rushing out the door to the car. As we're leaving, the nurse hands me a slip of paper with a phone number and a name on it. *Caroline.* She tells me the woman is the mother of a son with Down syndrome. I thank her over the cries of the babies and stuff the paper in my coat pocket.

"I feel like a Ping-Pong ball," Tom says, and I know exactly what he means.

We go from one thing to the next, back and forth, all day, every day, day in, day out, nighttimes, too. Sometimes I think of my old life, when we were a family of three. As I imagine it, I was always taking long baths, reading, and going to playdates with Carter. Memory can play cruel tricks. It seems as if I will be an old woman before the days of long baths and books return, I'm so far away from that life right now.

At seven months, this is our routine: Bennett wakes up at five a.m. I breast-feed him and he falls asleep again. Avery is up at six a.m.; Tom gets him, gives him a bottle, and puts him in the swing until seven a.m. By then, Bennett is up; Carter, too. We change diapers and clothes. Carter gets a chocolate milk. Tom brings in a stack of wood from outside and starts a fire in the woodstove. He drinks a cup of coffee, then heads down to the office.

I play with all the boys on the floor until breakfast, which is one-quarter cup rice cereal mixed with pears and a little yogurt. I feed Avery in the high chair and Bennett on the counter next to him in a bouncy chair. Carter eats Kix cereal and a bowl of yogurt. I clean up the kitchen, and change diapers. I no longer change the babies on the dryer, because they are both too wiggly. Instead, I use a bathroom towel on the floor.

I use cloth diapers with Diaperaps covers in the daytime; paper ones at night. I have ten wraps and two dozen Chinese prefolds that are hand-me-downs from a friend. Each morning I fill the washing machine half full of warm water and add two squirts of Dr. Bronner's lavender soap. When either of the babies has a dirty diaper, I toss it in the washer to soak. At the end of the day, I spin the cycle out, do another rinse, add All Free Clear, then run a final, hot wash. My last chore of the day is to toss the diapers and wraps in the dryer, so they will be ready for the morning.

I enjoy diapering the babies with cloth diapers. It's one of the things I'd hoped to do, before we knew we were having twins; one of the things I'd let go of that I'm reclaiming. I like the simplicity of it—it's just cloth and soap and water. I like the closeness of it; I have to change the babies more often than with the disposables, but it means I touch them more, too. And it gives me a peaceful feeling, knowing I can do this for them, particularly Avery. I want to do everything I can for him.

Next Bennett goes into the Exersaucer, and Avery goes on the floor for tummy time. I get Carter dressed for the day, and myself, too. I make a giant playpen for all the boys, using the couch as one side, the couch pillows as another, the overstuffed chair as the third, and a dining room chair tipped on its side for the fourth. They play inside the space, all together, me dropping in a new toy or changing a diaper as needed.

At nine a.m. the babies take their morning naps. Carter and I make a Play-Doh mess, or paint or color, until they wake up. I change diapers again and soon it is ten thirty. I feed Avery a bottle with one arm while nursing Bennett on the other side, burp both babies, switch sides, burp again, and it's back to the giant playpen.

When they tire of this, I put Bennett on the floor for his tummy time, which he uses to try to crawl. Avery goes in the Exersaucer, where he spins the spinner and clicks the clicker: he's excellent at the Exersaucer work. At eleven thirty it's mealtime again, vegetables and rice for all three boys. Then I clean up and do another round of diaper changes.

After lunch we go outside for some fresh air. Carter helps me push the stroller, or holds my hand, or wanders ahead, looking at rocks. This is the sweetest part of the day, when everyone seems content, me included. It's the fold on a page of paper; the front half is the morning, which we have already seen, the back half is the afternoon, which has not yet come. And we walk along our little lane in the woods, hearts and bodies and minds aligned in a straight path down the middle.

After our walk I give the babies a bath. I twist the knobs and run a tiny stream of warm water. I put Bennett in first, who sits firmly like the Buddha on the rubber safety mat, buoyed by the baby fat around his tummy and on his little legs. Avery is next—he is a little wobblier and I keep my hand on his shoulder to steady him. Avery is leaner and longer than Bennett, but he, too, has a little Buddha belly. His shoulders are narrower than Bennett's, and his hair is thicker and darker. Bennett is still mostly bald.

Avery likes to pat the water and sometimes it splashes on his face. He doesn't cry; he just smiles through the drops falling from his long, wet eyelashes and continues splashing. Bennett is nervous in the tub. He doesn't like being naked, he distrusts the water with its shiny surfaces, its strange slipperiness, and he hates Avery's splashing. If he gets even a drop on his face, he turns red with anger and begins screaming. Before this happens, I turn them back to back, so Avery can play and Bennett can calm down.

When we were first imagining twins, I decided I'd never dress them the same. I wanted them to be individuals, and one way I could support that, I thought, was to choose clothes for them as if they were singletons. Later, after Avery's diagnosis, I received in the mail a gift that helped me rethink my strategy. The package was from my friend Kathy, a wonderful writer and quilter who had made two baby quilts for us. With them came a note explaining that while she usually makes the quilts for twins unique, this time she made them the same. She wanted to emphasize the things our babies share in common. So on occasion, in the same spirit, I sometimes dress the babies the same. But mostly, it's a matter of practicality. Though we have many matching outfits, I rarely have two of each clean at the same time. But Kathy's quilts are always around as reminders of her insight.

I spread two towels on the floor, using just one hand, still holding on to Avery's shoulder. I pull him out first, careful not to drip on Bennett, and sit him on a towel. He is very flexible and folds in two like a rag doll. It reminds me of a yoga posture called *bala-asana*, which means Child Pose, that I can only reach after a lot of stretching and maneuvering. It's Avery's favorite position, and sometimes I find him like this in his sleep.

Bennett comes out next, and I swaddle him in the towel. Then I turn back to Avery, who's still wet as I smear Aquaphor all over his skin, paying particular attention to where the rash was, and also to his feet and hands, which have a tendency to become papery. I diaper him and dress him in a long-sleeved cotton onesie that is blue with white stripes. I like the way the blue sets off Avery's eyes.

With Bennett, speed is key. The less time he's naked, the happier he is. I rub lotion on his bottom only, then diaper and dress him quickly, my hands moving in a blur across his little body, the measure of my days—I can diaper and dress this baby in a matter of seconds. Bennett wears blue, too, a shade that complements Avery's outfit.

By the time bath has ended it's two thirty p.m. and the babies are ready for more nursing and bottle-feeding. A half hour later they take an afternoon nap, which is the longer one and lasts until it's almost supper. Carter and I have our special time together in the afternoons. We play games, or practice saying and writing the alphabet letters. Sometimes we make cakes or pies or cookies. If I'm feeling tired, I try to convince Carter to take a nap with me; sometimes he will, but sometimes he says, very seriously, "No nap, Mommy. Not today."

When the babies wake, it's close to five p.m. I feed them a supper of oatmeal and prunes, applesauce, more yogurt, sweet potatoes. I clean up again, change them into bedtime diapers (paper). More Aquaphor lotion for both babies and saline nose drops for Avery to keep his breathing easy; sometimes Bennett needs the drops, too. Both babies go into little blue sleep sacks to keep them warm through the night. They play on the floor beneath the big window, watching the lights reflected in the glass, the swirling snow. By now, Tom is home, too, and they are excited and interested in him.

Bedtime begins. Avery is first and I feed him alone now, taking him in—his eyes that sparkle and twinkle. His skin, so soft. When I pull him close, he seems to melt into me. He asks so little of me, really—all the rest of it I put upon myself.

Next is Bennett, the baby who often reminds me of a grumpy old man. I feel as if I spend most of my time coaxing him into things—eating, bathing, playing. It's as if I'm a cheerleader, jumping up and down, doing cartwheels, spinning in circles: give me a *B*! Give me an *E*! Give me an *N*! You can do it! Go go go! Goooo, Ben! All to have him open one eye, peek at a cloud, and call the game for rain.

Finally it's Carter's turn. Each night I read him a story. His current favorite is *King Bidgood's in the Bathtub* by Audrey Wood. When it comes to the part when it says, "Trout, trout, trout," he laughs and laughs. "Trout is a fish, Mommy," he tells me. "There's a fish in the bathtub!" After the story, we brush teeth and say a complicated good-night prayer, which includes everyone in the blessing.

Tom and I eat dinner late, but alone and in the quiet of the night. While we eat, I finish my routine with the diapers. Afterward, we make the night bottles and wash the dishes and pick up the house, both of us working together with an easy rhythm, which is the cadence of our lives.


Avery loves the piano. When I prop him in the bowl of my lap, he becomes very quiet and takes quick, panting breaths. I'm a beginner. I know two songs, "As Time Goes By" and "Someone to Watch Over Me." When I was pregnant I'd play them over and over, end to end, so that it seemed as if I had a full repertoire.

The piano is a simple upright made of old dark wood. Some of the keys stick and it's missing one of the knobs that pulls the cover shut. It's a gift from Phyllis, who knew of my secret wish to learn; when she saw the piano at a garage sale, nearly abandoned, its keys stripped of their ivories, she thought of me. She brought it home and cleaned the wood, repaired the broken strings, glued on new ivory. She worked until, for the first time in years, the piano could be played. It was a surprise birthday gift. She gave me a song. A song, and a piano to play it on.

"It has a lovely tone," she said. "You never would have guessed, looking at it."

When I play, Avery balanced on my lap, I think about his left ear. I look at it and wonder about the failed hearing test. I have all sorts of theories—there was fluid in it from the C-section. Or the machine malfunctioned. It was simply a bad test. Or his ear canals were too small. He needed time to grow. These are my hopes. I think about them as I play, willing the notes to go into Avery's left ear. Because he loves it so, I believe he can hear.

My hopes are the notes of this song.

Carter has taken up the habit of singing "Happy Birthday to You," though it's unclear whose birthday it is, exactly. The lyrics, according to him, are: "Happy birthday to you, happy birthday to you, happy birthday, dear birthday, happy birthday to you." It gives the days a festive flair.

Today is the birthday of no more preemie bottles. I toss them in the trash. We're moving on to Gerber colored. It feels like a big step forward. The decision was not made lightly, or without loads of research by me. For a while, I was considering using glass bottles, because of the possible danger of chemicals from the plastic bottles or the disposable liners. But I won't be able to get the glass bottles unless I order them online. And I'm not confident that I can keep them sterile (mildly germaphobic, still), so I decide to go with the disposable plastic liners. It's not a perfect solution: there are so many threats to worry about, trouble in all directions. Sometimes I just feel like sticking my head in the sand.

A person could say, *Well, gosh, you have bigger things to worry about, don't you?* It's precisely because of the bigger things that I worry about the little things. Decisions like what sort of bottles to use are within my control. But more important, I feel like we are already at a disadvantage with Avery. I don't want to add to the challenges he's going to face in life. More, even, than with my other sons, it feels like I need to pay attention to the details with Avery.

I try not to fuss over him, try not to single him out, especially in front of Carter. I don't want to color his relationship with his brother—I want it to develop on its own, naturally. But I've noticed that Carter is especially protective of the babies. He bodychecks his little friends like a linebacker if they get too close. And he's particularly protective of Avery. I wonder about it until a phone call with Joyce, when she comes up with a possible solution.

"Do you think it's because of when Avery used to be on the monitor?" she suggests.


I haven't had the "talk" with Carter about Down syndrome that I meant to have. It doesn't seem relevant yet. I know he won't understand the genetics; I know the medical concerns will confuse him, or scare him. I don't want to bring up anything that will prejudice him against Avery, but I also feel as if I need to mention it, at least. So I try to talk about it with him in a way that I think he'll understand.

"Have you heard Mommy or Daddy say the words 'Down syndrome'?" I begin.

"Yes," he says.

"Did you ever wonder what those words mean?" I ask.

"No."

"Well, let's talk about it anyway. Mommy wants to talk about it, okay?"

"Okay," he says.

"It's like this: everyone is born exactly the way they are meant to be. Some people have red hair, some people have brown. Some are tall, some are short. Some people have blue eyes, some green. And everyone is born with a speed. Some people have a fast speed, some people go slower. Everyone has their own speed."

I look down at him and wonder if he understands. It's difficult to explain it to him when I can barely make sense of it myself.

I start again. "Down syndrome means Avery will probably have a slow speed. It means it may take him longer to grow big, and it may take him longer to learn new things. But if we let him take his time, and if we love him, he will be fine."

"Okay," Carter says.

"Do you understand?" I ask.

"I get it," Carter says.

"You do?" I ask, surprised.

"It's like Clifford," he says. "Little things grow big with love."

"Exactly," I say, surprised by how easy it sounds when Carter says it. Clifford, the big red dog who grew and grew, all because of one little girl's great love.

There's a line of reasoning that goes like this: Avery has extra genetic material in every cell of his body. That material isn't inert. It has an effect on him, and its presence should be counterbalanced with what's currently called Targeted Nutritional Intervention (TNI). I check my books: *Understanding Down Syndrome*; *A*

*Parent's Guide to Down Syndrome*; *Babies with Down Syndrome*. From the three, I piece together the sixty-year history of TNI: In the 1940s, a doctor named Henry Turkel created the U-Series, a combination of forty-eight vitamins, hormones, and enzymes that he believed improved the appearance and intelligence of children with Down syndrome. Forty years later, another doctor, Ruth Harrell, and her colleagues began a nutritional therapy program with children of various diagnoses, including Down syndrome. Their program consisted of megadoses of vitamins, minerals, and a thyroid supplement. Like Turkel, Harrel reported an improvement in physical appearance and intelligence.

More recently, Dixie Lawrence Tafoya, a mother of a daughter with Down syndrome, enlisted medical researchers and biochemists to help create a program similar to Turkel's, which she called MSB Plus and began maufacturing through a Canadian company, Nutri-Chem. In 1996, Tafoya left Nutri-Chem and began promoting a different product, which is marketed in the United States by International Nutrition, Inc. Her new formula is called NuTriVene-D, and consists of more than forty ingredients, including vitamins, minerals, amino acids, antioxidants, digestive enzymes, and fat supplements.

My three books reach the same conclusions about TNI—there is an effect caused by the trisomy, but what it is, exactly, is unknown. Each chromosome carries genetic information for hundreds of thousands of biochemicals; our bodies consist of millions of controlled, orderly chemical reactions. Introducing additional biochemicals, with the hopes of mitigating others, is a guessing game, at this point. More research needs to be done.

I Google "Nutrivene-D." I find the company's Web site and click on it. I'm taken to a blue-and-purple screen featuring photos of happy, smiling people. An American flag waves in the right-hand corner. I notice a toll-free number, and a "view shopping cart" button. It seems like a legitimate business. In fact, it seems like a high-end vitamin shop. There are products for autism and probiotics for women, but I have trouble finding information about Down syndrome.

There's a FAQ section, which I click on, where I find questions like "What is Down sydrome?" with an answer that covers the overexpression of genes. "What is Nutrivene-D?" is answered with the names for the products—the Daily Supplement, Daily Enzyme, and NightTime Formula—but it doesn't list the ingredients. At the end, there is the question, "Is Nutrivene a cure for Down syndrome?" and the answer is a clear no, though it promises a more alert, healthier baby.

And then I think about Avery's little bird mouth. His little body, his round tummy, his skinny legs. Long fingers, long eyelashes, the stars in his eyes. He's such a good eater. I could put anything in his bottle and he'd take it; in his mouth, he'd swallow it. I try to imagine crushing the pills and putting them in his milk; or slicing open a gelcap and dribbling the contents onto his tongue. Two times a day, maybe three. In each instance, wondering if it's okay. Hoping I'm not hurting him. Guessing at the millions of biochemical reactions going on inside of him, knowing I'm altering them, but not knowing how.

I can't do it.

My friend Claudia is mother to a trapeze-swinging six-year-old girl. One of the best things about Claudia is that she always has thoughtful and intuitive things to say. When I ask her about a problem in my life, she tells me to think about what my heart is saying. And if that message is unclear, she tells me, "Deciding *not to decide* is a valid choice, too. You can choose not to decide, for today."

That's the way I feel about NuTriVene-D. I think the ideas are right; we all agree that something is going on within the little bodies of our children that disrupts the normal flow. But I've read over and over again that our children are more like other children than they are different. I go online one more time and

Google "Down syndrome nutrition." I see *The Down Syndrome Nutrition Handbook: A Guide to Promoting Healthy Lifestyles*, by Joan E. Guthrie Medlen. It's from Woodbine House, a publisher I recognize from many of the other books I've read and liked. And Joan Guthrie Medlen, in addition to being a registered, licensed dietician, is mother to a son with Down syndrome. I order the book.

When it comes, it feels as if it was written by a good friend, from one mother to another. Medlen's philosophy matches my own, which is that healthy eating is a lifestyle choice, and what I like best about the book is that it encourages being together in the kitchen, and exercising as a family. For now, her book is our answer to TNI.

Though it's the middle of January, the breeze is warm and smells of pine. This warm winter wind is called a chinook. The cold eye of winter is green—the grass is greening, the cottonwoods and the wild rose have sprouted the green tips of buds, even the mountains are a carpet of evergreens with only a whisper of snow at the highest peaks. It's as if spring is here. Spring is the time for babies, and I think back to the last spring I was pregnant, when my plans and hopes were so new and green.

Since my shopping trip with my dad, I've been more willing to bring the babies out in public. We pack ourselves up in much the same way we did then, only I can manage it by myself now. Carter is in his car seat near the window, with extra sippies and cheese crackers. Carter decides who he wants to sit next to; he chooses Avery; my guess is because he cries less than Bennett. I put Avery in his carrier, then bring him out to the car; last is Bennett. I pack the diaper bag with extra diapers, extra wipes, baby crackers, bottles, and we are off.

Instead of the giant carts of the warehouse store, our supermarket has carts that resemble miniature cars. Carter gets in and pretends to drive; I wear Bennett in the front pack, face-in, and Avery rides in his carrier in the child seat, where I can smile at him or feed him a bottle if he fusses.

The grocery store is having a sale—thick cardboard crates in a pyramid at the front entrance, ten lemons for a dollar. At that price, our whole town will be eating lemons—lemon chicken, lemon tart, lemonade. I choose ten and move on, talking to Carter and the babies as we go without even realizing it, until I see the startled look of a fellow shopper, a bearded man in jeans and a plaid shirt, who hears me say, "Do we need eggs today?" I look down and push the cart past him.

I add bananas to the cart. Milk, cheese. Diapers, wipes. A roasting chicken for dinner. At the bakery, Carter is accustomed to getting a free cookie. The woman who's usually there is a wiry, thin blonde. She makes a point of telling me what a good boy Carter is. "The bakery lady knows," she says. "They don't think we see, but we see. We're like Santa. We know who's naughty and we know who's nice."

She's the mom of twins, too (she's one of the *twin people*), and always asks about the babies. She peers at us from behind the counter, where she's been decorating a white cake with pink flowers. "I love babies," she says with a sigh, putting the pouch of icing down.

"Oh, um-hmm," I say, distracted by the display case, where I notice a chocolate cheesecake and a custard-fruit tart, side by side. The cheesecake has swirls of chocolate and chocolate shavings on top. But the fruit tart has sliced kiwis and whole strawberries arranged in a pattern that looks like a flower. A delicious, yummy flower. I try to decide which one is prettier: the fruit is covered with a glaze, so it glistens, but the chocolate shavings are mounded in a very artful way.

"I'd've had even more babies," she says, "but I got too old."

I nod my head at her, *Yes. I understand*. Maybe I'll splurge. I could buy one, but how to choose? I bet the babies would like it. Maybe the fruit tart?

"If I didn't stop having babies," she says, "I'd have a retard. A Down's kid, one of the ones that drools all the time."

I lift my eyes from the display counter. She sticks out her tongue and jerks her head side to side. "You know," she says, smiling at me.

I'm stunned. I look at her closely, in disbelief. She nods, wanting me to agree with her, waiting for my laughter.

I don't understand. Didn't she know about Avery? In this small town, it's hard to keep a secret. Was she teasing me? Or was she serious? It's too much to figure out. Tears spring to my eyes and I whip the giant pretend-car shopping cart around and quickly push it down the nearest aisle, toward the checkout.

Carter thinks it's a game and says, "Wheee, Mommy, faster!"

*Oh, Carter.* I wonder if he saw what the woman did; I wonder if he heard what she said. I consider leaving without the groceries, my cart of lemons and milk, bananas and eggs. But it's easier to get to the car if we take the cart. I'm trapped, a baby strapped to me, a baby in an infant seat, a child. I hold all of them. I carry us all. I can't move quickly, or fleetly. I'm wide and cumbersome and obvious; I'm a slow-moving vehicle; I'm an easy target.

I breathe in, breathe out. I blink back my tears. We hurry through the checkout, and when we're safely in the car, I am flooded with the "what-I-should-have-saids." I should have told her, *This is what a baby with Down syndrome looks like. Isn't he beautiful?* Or I should have said, *I used to feel that way, too. I don't anymore.* Or even, *Don't be afraid.*

But I didn't. I stumbled and fled, slowly, clumsily. I don't know who I feel bad for—Avery, Carter, or me. I hate feeling like a failure, like I'm letting Avery down. Next time I'll be ready. Next time, I'll know what to say.

At home, a word comes to me: despair. I'm the woman with

the retarded son. It's a hurt so deep that I only look at it when I'm forced to. I tell Tom about our day and the woman behind the bakery counter. With him, it feels safe, even manageable.

In the kitchen, smashing bananas for the babies' afternoon snack, I say, "We can't use the word 'retarded' anymore."

"I agree," he says.

"I didn't understand how hurtful it was."

"I know," he says. "But there are lots of retarded people in the world—Avery isn't one of them. Avery is one of the least retarded people I know."

"You said it twice."

We're having lemon chicken for dinner. The chicken is five pounds, nine ounces. I rinse it under a stream of water from the tap, pat it dry with paper towels in the cool stainless steel of the kitchen sink, then put it in a roasting pan and sprinkle it with salt and pepper. I cut a lemon and stuff both halves inside the chicken, along with sprigs of lemon thyme and parsley, then drizzle olive oil over the breast meat and the drumsticks. It goes into a 325-degree oven for two hours or so, until the skin is golden and the juices in the pan are clear. I baked a chicken like this when Sarah's second baby was born, and another for Phyllis's fifth. Roast chickens are whole-house meals, because while they cook, your whole house smells like supper.

After our day, all I want to do is stay in our big bed and read poetry. Gather my children into me and protect all the things I love with the things I love. Tenderness, softness. Cloth diapers in the dryer, tumbling. Classical guitar on the CD. The lemon chicken roasting in the oven. This is all I have to give; this is all I know to do.

I find a poem in a book called *A New Path to the Waterfall* written by Raymond Carver near the end of his life. The poem feels like the answer I wished I'd given to the woman behind the bakery counter. I say the words over and over again, checking myself against the dog-eared book, until I know them by heart:

> ***Late Fragment***
> *And did you get what*
> *you wanted from this life, even so?*
> *I did.*
> *And what did you want?*
> *To call myself beloved, to feel myself*
> *beloved on the earth.*

# 10

❧

# Alphabet Soup

Fog creeps across the lake from the north and settles. I haven't been outside in four days. Bennett has been up since four a.m. whining and nursing; nothing pleases him. Avery has been crying, too; I don't know why. Maybe it's the changeable weather—the warm winds have blown themselves away, and now it's back to valley inversions and more winter. On the answering machine are messages from my mom, and from my dad's wife, Pam. I know they're concerned and want to help, but I don't have the energy to put sentences together.

I nurse Bennett and Tom gives Avery a bottle. Bennett is still fussing. I try to feed him cereal. I can see by his expression that it's too lumpy. I water it down with milk, but again, no good. It's begun to snow. The fire in the woodstove is out. It's cold. I don't know where to begin. I'm tired and I have a headache and there are too many things to do. I think I'll cook eggs for Tom and Carter and me, everyone likes eggs, but when I open the fridge a bottle of barbecue sauce falls out and breaks, splattering its rusty contents all across the floor.

My head is throbbing. Bennett is crying. I grab a cloth from the sink and bend down and begin wiping. Tom is talking to me, saying something about last night's meeting at the fire department. I crack like the pieces of the barbecue sauce bottle.

"The problem with you is that you hold everything in until

you snap and that's why people think you're moody." Then, "I wish you enjoyed your nights out more. It's a strain on all of us when you're away, and you come home upset every time. I mean, enough already."

I take Bennett from the high chair and put him in the Pack 'n Play, still crying. I take Avery and put him in the swing. Tom is watching me; Carter, too. No one says anything. My heart is beating fast and I feel nauseous. I don't like being this angry. I leave the room and crawl into Carter's bed, where I pull the covers over my head. I take long, slow breaths until my heartbeat slows. My head still hurts. I'm so tired.

A little while later, Tom comes in. "I'm so sorry," I say. "It's me who holds things in, then snaps. You're the only big person around so I took it out on you. It's not right. I'm sorry," I say.

"It's okay," he says softly. "You need to sleep. Get some rest. I'll take care of things for a while." He leans in and kisses me on the top of my head.


When I wake, the light has the weak slant of afternoon to it. My headache is gone. A fire glows in the woodstove, and a stack of split wood is piled neatly nearby. The kitchen floor has been washed. The toys have been put away, and the carpet has been vacuumed. But what I notice the most is the quiet. Tom has taken Carter and the babies outside, to play in the fresh snow. I pull on my coat and boots and join them.

The air is crisp and cold and fresh and feels like a brand-new start. The sun is out, and the snow is a rainbow of colors. I go to Tom and hug him.

"Thank you," I say.

"No problem."

I find the babies, bundled and strapped in the stroller. I kiss Avery, then Bennett. And then Carter, who is crunching his feet in the snow as a demonstration for his brothers, who are spellbound by his skills. I try to kiss him, too, but he turns away from me. It's the first time I remember him doing this. I'm filled with sadness, and regret. My boy. He's growing up so fast.

These are the things Avery can do: lift his head, roll, sleep, feed himself a bottle. This is what he can't do: crawl. I add it to the growing list of questions I have about Avery in my little spiral notebook: "Loose/tense muscles? Spine curve, vocalizations/hearing, balance? Passive versus active—his natural personality, or DS?" My problem is that I don't know whom to ask. The more I read, the more it seems there is only one person who has the answer: Avery. He holds the key in the palm of his tiny, creased hand.

I put him in the Exersaucer and pull it next to me. Bennett is sitting in my lap, trying to type at the computer keys. I absentmindedly push his hands out of the way, trying to work quickly, opening one of the sites I bookmarked earlier: the NDSS, which is the organization that sent the new parents' information packet. The computer screen changes to a blue, tan, and red home page, then pictures of babies, kids, teens, and adults appear. Quotes beneath the changing photos read, *that she will be able to make her own decisions and have others believe in her* and *for my son to have a fulfilling life* and *that people with Down syndrome will be seen as people and are no longer labeled* and *that all parents will know it's not the end of the world to have a child with Down syndrome.*

Bennett coos when he sees the babies and tries to touch the screen; I grab both of his wrists with my left hand and continue reading: *I hope our son grows up to be a contributing member of our community* and *that children and parents will be given hope for the future.*

I examine each photo as if it held important clues. I see a young girl blowing bubbles, and I remember the first time I blew bubbles with Carter—a warm spring day, and we sat on a blanket in the grass. Next is a photo of a young man playing guitar, and I think maybe Avery should play the guitar. A picture of a boy looking at a card that reads, "Happy Birthday, We love you, Dad and Mom."

I study haircuts and clothes, toys and activities. I see a boy in a kayak on a lake and think, *We could kayak*. I see a child playing with a Mr. Potato Head doll and think, *We should get a Mr. Potato Head*. A little girl in a blue ballet outfit; another in a red one. Bennett is unhappy, so I switch the babies around—Avery comes into my lap, and Bennett goes into the Exersaucer. He swats at the blue-and-red steering wheel, then gets his arm stuck. I free him, and pat his head.

The NDSS sponsors several events each year: a gala auction, a spring luncheon and boutique, a golf outing. Their main event is the Buddy Walk, which takes place in the fall. I notice a bunch of kids all wearing Buddy Walk T-shirts, and I look closely at them, trying to guess who has Down syndrome and who doesn't. The Buddy Walk is a day of fund-raising and awareness held concurrently in more than three hundred affiliate locations across the country.

I'm interrupted by the phone. It's my sister, Glynnis. "What size are the babies?" she asks. I can barely hear her. "Is twelve months okay?"

"Sure. What's going on? Where are you?"

"Shopping," she says. She tells me about her migraines, and the hormone shots she's been giving herself to get ready for her first round of in vitro at the end of March. The last time I saw her, Carter was just a baby. She whispered to him, singing a song so softly I could barely make out the words. "You are my sunshine, my only sunshine," she sang, just like my mother used to sing to us.

And now, she's calling me on her cell phone from a sale rack in the baby aisle, buying things for my children because she's not sure if she'll ever have children of her own. Again, I'm reminded of my life, my burden that is not a burden—my children, an abundance simply given to me.

We hang up and I remember the slip of paper from the nurse at the county health department. I go to my coat and search the pockets until I find it, crumpled but intact. I call and introduce myself to the woman on the other end of the line. Caroline, mother to Robby. That's all I know about her; and yet, I ask Caroline about Avery's crawling. "Did it take Robby a long time to crawl?"

She says she doesn't remember any problem, but asks if I'd like to come to her house to talk. I say yes, and we make arrangements.


The next afternoon, I leave Carter and the babies with Tom and drive to the address, which is a new house in the golf course development. All morning, I'd fretted over what to wear and what to bring. I settled on jeans and a green blouse that I hoped looked clean and casual; I'd decided to give her a copy of the book I edited about parenthood. One of my favorite essays was written by a mother of a child with learning disabilities. As I ring the bell, I have butterflies in my stomach.

The door opens and she's younger than her voice sounded, younger than I imagined. She's slim and pretty, with brown hair and a bright smile. She invites me inside her spotless home, to a room with vaulted ceilings, cream carpeting, and a matching leather family room set.

"Robby is home from school," she tells me. "I'll get him." She disappears down a hallway to the left and returns holding the hand of a boy Carter's size, with blond hair and blue eyes. I suck in my breath. He's the spitting image of Avery, if Avery were six years older.

He's not particularly interested in me, but his mom tells him, "Say hello, Robby." He does, grudgingly. Then he motions that he wants to go back to his room. His mom bends down to his ear and whispers something, and he nods. He goes down the hall and returns, dragging a wooden castle behind him into the family room, knights and horses in a bundle beneath his arm. I have an overwhelming urge to give him a hug.

"Is it okay if I play with him?" I ask Caroline.

"Sure," she says.

I kneel down on the floor, take a plastic toy horse, and tentatively begin. I gallop the horse over to the tower, then neigh. Robby laughs. I gallop away, and he laughs again. He gets a horse and begins chasing me. I neigh and run away, moving my horse around the tower. He turns quickly, catching me. I laugh. It reminds me of playing with Carter.

He asks me something, motioning with his hands, and I have trouble understanding what he means. I look to his mom, who says, "He wants to know if you want a cookie."

"Is it okay?" I ask.

"Sure," she says.

"Yes, I'd love a cookie," I tell Robby. I turn to ask his mom if he understands, but he's already racing into the kitchen, where he pulls out a stool at the breakfast bar and pats the stool next to him, indicating I should join him.

Caroline gets me and Robby each an Oreo and a glass of milk. Sitting, sipping, eating. He dunks. I dunk. When we finish eating, he asks his mom something and again, I don't understand. She explains. "He wants to know if he can watch his cartoons." She tells him yes, and gets him settled on the couch.

While he's busy, she and I sit on stools at the kitchen counter. She tells me she was very young when she had Robby. He was born early and stayed in the NICU. I nod and tell her my twins came early, too. She's a nursing student and will graduate soon. She doesn't plan on having any more kids—I want to ask why, but to press the point seems rude. Instead, I ask about crawling. She says Robby used to scoot around all over; she doesn't remember him ever having a problem. She asks if I've called CDC.

"No," I admit, "not yet."

"You should call them," she tells me. "They'll help."

The cartoon is over and Robby wants Doritos. Caroline tells him he can have three. He goes to the cupboard, takes out the bag, and stuffs three into his mouth. Then he takes three more in his hand.

"No, Robby," she says. "Three means three." He sulks. I've seen this all before at my house, over any number of things. I admire her firmness and her resolve. To diffuse the situation, she asks Robby if he wants to play a song on the piano.

He shakes his head no.

She asks if he wants to tell me about riding his horse.

Again, no.

She asks if he wants to play castles.

Still no.

As a last resort, she asks if he wants to read a story.

His eyes light up.

"Go get the book from your school bag," she says.

He does, and returns, settling himself into the overstuffed chair. Pats for me to sit next to him, then opens the book to the first page, to the words "I can. . . ." I think he means for me to read it, so I begin. Caroline stops me. "Let him do it," she says gently. I'm surprised, and shocked, and I can't remember when I've been so excited.

He speaks in thick but unmistakable syllables. It's a struggle for him, I can tell, but it becomes clear to me that he understands what he's seeing, and what he's saying. I begin to cry. Tears leak out of my eyes and I think, *Well, who needs help here?* I'm overcome with happiness, and hope, and love for this little boy whom I only just met but feel as if he's my own. Caroline pats my shoulder and nods with empathy. "I know," she says, "I know. It's pretty awesome."

The book ends. I tell Robby that I think he's terrific and I ask if I can give him a hug. He nods yes, reverting back to the signs and gestures that he seems the most comfortable with. I have to get home to my own family, but I don't want to leave. I want to stay here forever, in this moment, Robby reading to me, *I can, I can, I can.*

The number for the CDC is in a pink, purple, red, and orange brochure that's been on the fridge since we got home from the NICU. Today, I unfold it and read the listings: Evaluation and Diagnostic Services. Autism Spectrum Disorder Evaluations. NICU Follow-up Screening Clinics. Early Childhood Screenings. Family Education and Support. Helping parents and children learn new skills. "A private, non-profit organization funded in part through the Montana Department of Health and Human Services, serving seven counties in western Montana. Degrees in child development, special education, pediatric therapy or related field."

I make the phone call and reach an answering machine. I state my purpose: "My name is Jennifer Groneberg and my son Avery has Down syndrome and I don't know what to do for him." This is the first time I've said it like that—the simple, unadorned facts. As I speak, I try to keep my voice even and unemotional, but near the end, my façade cracks and the *I don't know what to do for him* part comes out in a rush. I hang up and wait for a return phone call. When it comes, I try my best to seem confident and calm.

The day of our first appointment arrives, and I bundle up the babies and Carter for the short drive to the highway to meet Brittney, who drives a Subaru. I'd thought about giving her directions over the phone, or drawing her a map and sending it to her in the mail, but there are very few road signs, and even if you think you know the way, it's easy to get lost. We agree instead to meet at the highway, so she can follow me home.

I check my rearview mirror often, making sure she's behind me. As we drive, I imagine seeing what she sees. The twisty road. So many trees. The blue water of the lake peeking through the woods. The rock outcroppings. More trees, and houses that I know are there, tucked way back, but that can't be seen. The road rises, up and up. I turn into what must look like a wall of trees, but it's our driveway. Up again. She's still there. I park and begin getting the kids out. She pulls in alongside me.

"Wow," she says. "I never would have found it on my own."

I look over at her. She seems young, fresh out of college. She's wearing low-rise jeans, thick-soled shoes, funky black glasses. She has a red stripe in her dark brown hair. I wonder what draws people to this kind of career. I want to tell her not to work too hard. Play at life, fall in love, have babies of her own.

"It's really something out here. Like another world," she says. "I bet it's pretty quiet."

I smile at her. You can tell a lot about people by their first reactions to the drive out to our house. Sometimes it's awe; other times, people want to know, right away, how to get back to the main road. But today, I'm cautious. This isn't an ordinary situation, and no matter how hard I try, I can't forget it. I feel as if she's here to judge me, which makes me cautious.

"Do you ever get lonely?" she asks.

"No," I say, the only answer. I won't give her any reply that has a hole in it.

She fumbles with something in the back of her car, and I begin taking the baby carriers out. She carries her own things, a giant black bag and a purse and a thick binder filled with papers. We make our way into the house, where the radio is playing softly and soup cooks in the Crock-Pot. The toys are all put away, the carpet vacuumed, the floor swept. This is, perhaps, the biggest deception—my house is never this tidy without a lot of work. I put each baby in his high chair, and ask if she minds if we eat lunch first. It's a test of sorts: I hope she'll share a meal with us.

When Tom and I were first married, and we lived on the wide-open plains of eastern Montana, I was introduced to the notion of "neighboring" by a woman named Grace. Grace wore her white hair pinned in a bun on top of her head. Her gray eyes blinked out through big round glasses. She drove her Lincoln Town Car too fast and was often found in the ditch, calmly waiting for someone to pass by on a tractor and pull her out. She began every phone call in the middle of a conversation, saying things like, "Is it hot enough for you?" or "When do you think we're going to get some rain?"

It always took me longer than it should have to realize who was calling, and the uncertainty of it made me feel a little topsy-turvy, which was the perfect frame of mind for being around Grace. She held on to the old-fashioned idea of neighboring, which meant that she expected you to drop by from time to time, and when you did, it was best if you planned to break bread. Serving Brittney soup is perhaps the truest thing about the day—this is who we are, this is what we believe. If you're going to be a part of it, this is where we start. We'll break bread.

Brittney agrees to have lunch, but she's unsure where to sit. Maybe she's nervous, too. I tell her to sit in the middle, where the view is the best. The lake is steel gray with little whitecaps rising and falling. Low clouds hang over the water and you can't see very far; even the lake is guarded, not revealing too much of itself. I set out the bowls and the spoons and the bread and we begin eating. She doesn't ask me about Avery; instead, she tells me about herself. As she speaks, her posture changes, from straight and upright to a casual slouch. She says she loves kids, though she doesn't have any of her own. She's an aunt, though, and spends lots of time with her brother's children.

Her title in the brochure is Family Support Specialist, an occupation I'm not familiar with, and I find myself asking in as many subtle ways as I can, "But what is it you do, again?" She's brought a stack of papers for me to read and sign, one with the title "Description of Service Deliverer." It explains that Brittney will offer education and support, generally provided in our home on a weekly basis. She'll implement a plan designed to promote the developmental needs of Avery. She'll show me strategies and teaching techniques, and help me obtain and coordinate necessary resources. A thought comes to me: *I wonder if she can help me figure out our health insurance.*

I go through the rest of the papers. One explains that the CDC "strengthens families to promote the development and well-being of individuals with developmental disabilities or who are at risk for developmental delay." I have no idea what that means. Another page is a sort of family bill of rights that says each family is unique, each child is unique, and the child's family is the primary member of the team—involvement in services must always be the family's choice. I still have no idea who the team is, or what the services are. There's a Service Agreement, and a procedure for discontinuing services—if the child grows up or moves; if I fail to participate in follow-through to which I agree; if I keep fewer than 50 percent of my appointments, or miss three consecutive visits over a six-month period; if I misuse CDC funds.

I begin getting a knot in my stomach. Grievance procedures, mandated reporting. I skim through the rest of the language, peeking at it with one eyeball. I don't have anywhere else to turn, so I sign at the *X*s. She gives me more information to read and a DVD about Down syndrome to watch. If I have any questions, she'll be back in a week, or I can always call. Despite my doubts, I find myself liking Brittney. At the end of the meal, she helps me clear the dishes from the table and offers to help load them into the dishwasher.

After everything is cleaned up, she asks me about Avery. I pull out my notebook and read my questions about loose muscles, the curve of his spine, vocalizations and hearing. I don't think she'll have the answers; and really, there's just one thing I want help with. When will Avery crawl?

She doesn't know. She tells me there are people who might, though; maybe she can set up some appointments for me. She tells me it begins with an evaluation by our doctor. We get a referral from him to see a specialist. Then the specialist does an evaluation, and we go from there. "Is this okay with you?" she asks.

It seems like it'll be a very long time before I get the answers I need, if at all. But I'm willing to try. I say yes. "Should I make another appointment with our doctor, then?" I ask, already beginning to worry about the extra cost.

"If you've seen your doctor recently, like for well-checks, you might just need to call your doctor's nurse, who can help you with the referral. It's a piece of paper, like a prescription, for therapy."

I nod, okay. "One more thing?" I ask. "We have terrible health insurance for the kids. Is that something you might help us with?"

"Let me check into it," she says. "I'll bring some information next time I come out."

In my little notebook, I begin making a list of abbreviations for the different kinds of therapies. The first is Early Intervention (EI), which is a general term that includes family education, counseling and home visits, speech pathology and audiology, vision testing and support, physical therapy, occupational therapy, and any health services necessary to enable an infant or toddler to benefit from the other services. It also includes coordination of diagnostic services and help with transportation, if necessary.

Fine motor skills are body movements that use small muscles, like picking up a Cheerio and putting it in a container, or pouring liquid from one cup into another. Occupational therapy (OT) helps a child's many systems work together—the muscles, the skeleton, and the nervous system—and all the ways they coordinate, including balance, perception, reflexes, and the development of fine motor skills.

Gross motor skills include body movements that use the

large muscles—for example, sitting, crawling, walking, or climbing. Physical therapy (PT) activities are designed to increase gross
motor skills, prevent or alleviate movement dysfunction, and to
build strength, range of motion, coordination, and endurance.

Expressive language is the ability to communicate through
speech, writing, augmentative devices, or gestures. Receptive
language is the receiving and understanding of language. Speech
therapy (ST) builds communication skills in both expressive language and receptive language, and encourages oral motor development for such tasks as speaking and eating.

I also write down any acronym I come across and its meaning. Some of the terms I know from firsthand experience: ABR
(Avery's failed hearing test at the chapel), CDC (Brittney's office),
FSS (Brittney's job title), and SSI (the supplemental income we
didn't qualify for).

I add some of the abbreviations for terms describing children
with differences in learning styles or developmental delays, including: AD (attachment disorder), ADD (attention deficit disorder), ADHD (attention-deficit/hyperactivity disorder), AS
(Asperger's syndrome), and ASD (autism spectrum disorders). I
learn that some children have more than one diagnosis, and that
others don't fit neatly into any of these categories, so they have
their own acronym: PDD-NOS (pervasive developmental disorder, not otherwise specified).

The DVD Brittney left for me is called *Down Syndrome: The
First 18 Months.* I put the babies down for their naps, take out
canary yellow Play-Doh for Carter, and put on the show to watch
while we work. I take a clump and make a ball in the palm of my
hand. I push the ball onto the kitchen counter, rolling it into a log.
I shape the log into a C. "Now you," I say to Carter.

The words "A Story: Just a Boy" come on the television
screen, followed by images of a beautiful little boy drawing
on the cement with chalk. The boy and his mother in a swimming pool. A newborn baby wearing a little white cap, just like

Bennett's. The baby growing into the boy from the earlier photos. Holding hands, with his mother, his sister. Holding the chalk on the cement again, as if the story has looped back to the beginning, but now you know this family, and their boy with Down syndrome.

Next is "47 Chromosomes," a segment by Dr. Allen C. Crocker, Program Director for the Institute of Community Inclusion at the Children's Hospital in Boston. He's a kind, grandfatherly type, and as he explains the science of Down syndrome, I think, *That's the doctor we should've had for Avery.*

Carter makes a *C* and I move on to another ball, and log, and make an *A.* "You too," I say to him.

The "Finding Out" stories begin, and women come on the screen talking about the diagnosis of Down syndrome and what it meant to each of them. One woman seems as if she's about to cry, and I wonder how long it takes before you can talk about it *without* feeling like you're about to cry.

I watch and listen, playing with Carter, making bright yellow letters. The softness of the dough and its familiar, comforting smell; Carter's careful concentration—these things make me feel brave and I'm able to absorb more information than I have at any one time previously. The DVD goes over newborn health care, and a woman comes onscreen. The caption identifies her as Joan Guthrie Medlen, who wrote the book about Down syndrome and nutrition. It feels like I've just seen a friend on TV. I stop rolling Play-Doh and watch as she describes how to breast-feed a baby with Down syndrome. I think about Avery, and how we didn't have that experience, and a little wave of regret washes over me. I wish I'd seen this DVD earlier; maybe it might have helped.

I take up another ball, and roll it in the palm of my hand, then another, helping Carter finish his name. A new segment begins called "A Story: William's Heart." A biracial couple has a son with Down syndrome and also a heart condition. As they tell their story, they make it clear that their trouble was with the heart problem, not with Down syndrome. I remember Bennett's surgery, and I believe I understand their feelings.

The DVD continues, with more information from parents and doctors. A geneticist, MDs, a professor at the Down Syndrome Educational Trust. One woman has a British accent, like Dr. Anne. There are speech pathologists, an otolaryngologist, a physical therapist. Information about mealtimes and dental care and how to schedule therapies. More parent interviews. The statistics in my binder from the hospital say that Down syndrome affects all races, across all walks of life. So far, the families in this DVD have all been different, and unique, and completely unremarkable. Mothers, fathers, siblings. It could happen to anyone. It happened to us.

I'm left with the idea that our life is doable. That it's okay; that we'll be okay. I accept the feeling quietly, rolling a Play-Doh ball in the palm of my hand, then another, helping Carter fashion them into snowmen—a mother and a father, a boy, two babies. I marvel at it: our family, beautiful and whole, each of us, glowing like the sun.

Brittney has brought rosemary–olive oil bread from a bakery called the Knead, and her supervisor, Carolyn, has homemade pasta salad. I made vegetable soup with pasta shaped like the letters of the acronyms and abbreviations in my notebook— homemade alphabet soup. Carolyn is mom to two young girls, and has past experience working with children with Down syndrome. Both women are here to begin the evaluation process for Avery, which we start right after lunch. And there's good news: Brittney has information on a statewide children's insurance plan for families who aren't covered by Medicaid, and she thinks we'll qualify. All I have to do is complete the paperwork.

After lunch, we use the Early Learning Accomplishment Profile (E-LAP) scoring booklet for children functioning in the birth-to-thirty-six-month developmental age range. Carolyn, Brittney, Avery, and I sit on the carpeting on the floor. Brittney pulls toys from her big black bag; Carolyn makes checkmarks on the booklet, asking questions when she's not sure, things like, "Have you ever seen Avery stack one block on top of another, like this?" or "Have you noticed him searching for a toy that's been hidden, like this?" Brittney demonstrates, showing me what Carolyn means, and tries to get Avery to participate.

He's reluctant; it's almost nap time and he's getting sleepy. Bennett thinks it looks like fun and wants to play, too. I let him try a bit, but when it's Avery's turn, he fusses. I think I shouldn't have Bennett around if we do this again, but singling out Avery doesn't feel right, either. I don't want to push Bennett away, simply because he doesn't have Down syndrome. And Bennett will be a part of Avery's life long after these two women have gone; it's important that I preserve and protect their feelings for each other. I decide that next time, I'll try to match the test items with our own toys so that we have two of everything—the blocks, the pegs, the cups with Cheerios in them—so that Bennett can participate, too.

The test is divided into sections: gross motor, fine motor, cognitive, language, self-help, and social/emotional. The achievements are scored as + or -, and are graded by age-appropriateness. Carolyn begins with tasks she can see Avery has already mastered, which feels good. When she gets to the things he can't do, it hurts. My pride turns to defensiveness and I think things like, *Who cares that he can't push up on his hands and knees and rock? What a useless skill! Or, Wait, what about his adjusted age?* Then, *Of course he can't sit down from standing without holding on. He can't even crawl! That's why I called!* And, *Carter couldn't do that either at ten months.*

On the fine motor portion, we do better. Avery rings a bell. He picks up a cube using the palmar grasp. He holds, bites, and chews a cookie. He uncovers a toy hidden beneath a scarf—which

I didn't know he could do. Carolyn asks me if he can poke. I don't know. Brittney demonstrates: a finger poking through a hole. Again—finger, hole. This seems ridiculous to me. What kind of skill is the *poke*?

The Cognitive section causes more trouble: Does he imitate sounds? Shake his head no? Can he poke? *Now we're repeating ourselves*, I think, determined to teach Avery to poke before the next evaluation. On the Language section, and the next one, Self-Help, we do better: He responds to yes and no. He knows his name. He holds his own bottle. He can find his feet with his hands, he can touch his nose with his fingers.

Finally we're on the last segment, Social-Emotional. Avery can smile. He can pat, he vocalizes to a mirror. He responds to verbal requests, and will do simple nursery rhymes like "Itsy Bitsy Spider." He repeats a laughed-at performance. He understands no. He gives a toy to an adult on request. He wants to be near adults, and shows the emergence of stranger anxiety. Avery's evaluation in this category puts him at the developmental level of a fourteen-month-old, though his adjusted age is seven months.

I think about what our family doctor said, when I was so proud of Avery's rolling. I wonder if he's right—Avery will inevitably fall behind, and break my heart, again and again and again. It doesn't feel true. Even though Avery has done well on this part of the test, I can see that it's not the true measure of him. The papers and their letters and the yes-or-no answers aren't the whole story. They don't capture Avery's gentle, easygoing nature. They don't mention how he sucks his foot. There's no place to check off how he opens and closes his fist, which Tom calls "the sound of one hand clapping." The way his chin quivers when he cries; the stars in his eyes. The most important things don't fit on any form; they are not quantifiable, or able to be gauged. But they count—they are the measure of love.

# 11

### ❧

# Taxi Rides

Avery is perched on top of a giant blue exercise ball wearing what I call his frowny face. Every muscle is scrunched into a grimace and he's about to begin howling. Holding him steady, nonplussed by his theatrics, is Wendy. She's rolling Avery around on top of the ball by supporting his legs. He has to maintain his balance by using his waist, the core of his body's strength, and he's not happy about it.

"This will help him get stronger," she says cheerfully, "and that will help him crawl." She guides my hands to Avery's legs, and shows me how to move the ball myself. "There," she says, "just touch him gently. You're cueing the muscles to act, reminding them. Then let Avery do the work." We roll him left, then right, forward, then back. All the while Avery's frowny face is firmly in place.

"Just think how happy he'll be when he can crawl," Wendy offers.

She's right. Avery's frowny face will disappear when he can get about on his own.

Wendy is Avery's pediatric physical therapist. She's my age or a bit younger, with shoulder-length brown hair and a thin, muscular build. She feels wholesome and good for you, like apples. She became a physical therapist because when she was small, maybe Carter's age, her aunt was in a terrible accident that left her requiring months of rehabilitation. Wendy saw her while she was in the hospital, and the visit left an impression. She knew that someday she wanted to help people heal their bodies, too, especially children.

She asks more of Avery than I do, pushes him harder than I would. At times, it's difficult for me to watch. I want to say, "Enough! He's just a baby! Stop!" but I hold my tongue. My need to help Avery is greater than my need to comfort him, and I believe Wendy is helping Avery.

Wendy teaches me as she's teaching Avery. She demonstrates a posture or body movement that Avery could be learning, that I might watch for at home. And then she gently places her hands over mine, showing me how to hold Avery to support his budding skills. For instance, my worry over Avery's crawling. Bennett had been crawling for weeks; Avery seemed to want to crawl, but all he could manage was a sort of full-body stretch, as if he were an Olympic ski jumper extending all his limbs to get maximum air. Sometimes, as he did the ski-jumper pose, he'd shriek, a combination of enthusiasm and exasperation.

I tried all sorts of things to help Avery move beyond the ski jump into actual crawling: hand-over-hand movements, modeling, putting him on my own body as I crawled so he could feel how it was supposed to go. Nothing worked. Left to his own devices, he resorted back to the ski jumper, and his shrieks began to have a more frustrated tone—prompting a chain of events including Caroline, then the CDC, then Brittney, our family doctor's nurse, and finally, Wendy.

Wendy took one look at the ski-jumper position and put Avery on the big blue exercise ball, explaining that he needs to build up his trunk muscles, so that he'll have the core body strength necessary to move all his limbs in the coordinated pattern crawling requires. She also shares with me pages from *Gross*

*Motor Skills for Children with Down Syndrome*. My homework is to read the chapter we are currently working on, and come to our next meeting with any questions.

At the end of our half-hour session, Wendy stops working a bit early, to allow time to hold Avery, to love him and kiss him and tell him what a good boy he is. She says this is so he won't learn to hate therapy. But there's such honesty to her hugs, so much enthusiasm in her voice as she praises him, that I think there's more to it. I think she loves each of her students, just as the best nurses in the NICU loved each of the tiny babies.


Nifty Thrifty is a secondhand store in town that supports, in part, programs and activities for adults with disabilities. Before becoming Avery's mom, I used to shop there on occasion, when I was working on the newsletter, and now I have a nagging urge to go there with Avery. I think I'm hoping for something to happen, for some guidance, like back in the beginning, with Sandy B.'s *meaningful hug* and the *woo-woo cards*. I've been on my own for a while, and I want to check in. I have the idea that this place is Avery's, and that here I might get some answers. I feel so silly about it that I don't even tell Tom; I merely swing by the store one day on my way home from physical therapy.

Bells jingle as I haul the car seat, with Avery inside, through the glass front door. On our right, there is a checkout counter and cash register. There, a young woman sits on a stool, a baby in a car seat at her feet. She sees Avery and me, brightens, then smiles.

"How old is your baby?" she asks.

"Ten months."

"He's small, then," she says as she notices, more curious than accusing.

"He has Down syndrome," I say carefully.

"Did you breast-feed him?" she asks.

"No." There, I said it, surprising myself. I don't feel apologetic or embarrassed.

"Me neither. I really tried, but it was too hard," she says, and looks to me for sympathy.

I nod in agreement.

"Does your baby ever sleep?" she asks.

"Yes, he's a very good sleeper," I say. It's true.

"My baby never, ever sleeps. I mean, he sleeps in the day, but he's up all night. I am so tired."

Again, I nod to this young mother, hungry for someone to talk to. I'm hungry, too, I realize, for talk with other mothers about all the things that go with having a baby, topics that have nothing to do with Down syndrome, like first smiles and little coos and teething and what to do for diaper rash.

A few people putter around us, shopping. On a table near the counter are mason jars filled with buttons, and I'm reminded once more of my work for the newsletter. One of the jobs for people at the organization's activity center was to cut buttons from worn clothing, to save and resell. During a break between interviews, I noticed a man wearing thick glasses hunched over a different table, alone, drawing crayon circles on a white sheet of butcher paper. His right hand, which was long and elegant, circled and circled the page in what seemed like one fluid motion. I'd been mesmerized by it, until he stopped and banged his hand on the table. A woman from the buttons came over, took away the sheet of paper, replaced it with a fresh one, and the man began his motions again. On her way back to the button table, the woman threw the circles in the trash.

"Can I keep that?" I spoke up, pointing to the paper.

"Why would you want it?" she asked.

"I like it," I said.

"Sure, go ahead."

I brought the paper home and kept it above my desk for a while. Each circle was exactly the same as the one before it, and the one after it, and no two circles touched. The colors changed gradually in families of shades—blues to greens to purples to reds. I used to look at it and try to imagine what this man saw through his thick lenses, wonder how it felt to be him. I don't know what happened to the paper. I haven't thought of it, or the man and his circles, in a long while.

The young mother brings me back from my memories to the present day. "Have you started solids yet?" she asks.

I nod.

"Is your baby a good eater?" she asks.

"Yes. He feeds himself, most of the time," I say. I can see her deflate a little; I shouldn't have told her about the feeding-himself part—it's not like I had anything to do with it. He taught himself.

"You're so lucky," she says, and I think for a moment she's making fun of me, but no, she means it. From her point of view, having a baby who sleeps and eats well makes me lucky.

"Sure," I say.

As if on cue, Avery begins fidgeting. I need to get going. I don't know what I expected. There was no ticker-tape parade when we entered, no balloons and confetti falling from the ceiling. I take one last look around at the jars of buttons, the wall of straw wreaths, the racks of color-coded clothes. Shoes in a line, littlest to biggest. Scarves at the checkout, and a dull gold necklace and a basket full of eyeglasses. Part of me is still looking for clues, one last time. I pick up Avery, ready to go. Being his mom doesn't hurt so much, today.

"Didn't you need something?" the young mother asks from her stool.

"I guess not," I say, feeling like a goof. "Have a good day."

After weeks of hormone shots that left bruises scattered across her thighs like violets—dark blue and purple, yellow and green—my sister is pregnant. For the last step of the in vitro procedure, she was strapped into a contraption that held her upside down for the implantation. Our mother was there. They all said a prayer over Glynnis as she hung suspended in midair.

When my sister called to tell me about it, all I could picture was the *Vitruvian Man*, a drawing with accompanying notes created by Leonardo da Vinci. In it, a human figure is drawn in two superimposed positions—in one pose, the arms are wide apart and the legs are together; in the other, the arms are raised, and the legs are apart. The figure is simultaneously inscribed in a square, symbolic of our material existence, and a circle, which represents our spiritual life. The *Vitruvian Man* is a *cosmografia del minor mondo* (cosmography of the microcosm), in which the workings of the human body are an analogy for the workings of the universe. In my mind, my sister's Vitruvian man has been spun like a wheel of fortune.

At the follow-up appointment, her doctor kissed her on the head and said it wasn't every day that you witness a miracle. I think of Glynnis, and the baby growing inside of her, and the cosmography of the microcosm. Cells multiplying. Chromosomes joining, then dividing. The genetic blueprint. A road map of life, in fine blue lines.

I envision all that she has ahead of her—unwrapping her baby, and recognizing her own long fingers in his. Sweet kisses on dewy-soft skin. Watching her son sleep on his father's chest, or in her arms. Little grunts, tiny smiles, the first coo, a laugh that is so beautiful you laugh, too. I missed so much of this with Avery, irreplaceable moments lost to sadness and worry. It didn't have to be this way. I wish I had known better. I wish I had known that all I had to do was love him.


"Mommy, this color is called ketchup," Carter tells me, as we are sitting at the dining room table. He's drawing pictures and I'm feeding Avery. Bennett is trying to walk tippy-toed around the chair. I marvel at his natural ability, and also think back to Carter. My two sons, early walkers. Physically coordinated. Able. And then there's Avery the ski jumper. Wendy says he'll crawl when he's ready. She says not to worry. He's getting stronger each week. "Soon," she says, patting my hand. "Soon."

It's raining again, a late spring storm of big round drops that mesmerize the babies. I move them to the carpet near the window. Avery reaches for a yellow race car, stretching himself out to his full ski jumper, and begins chirping, not unlike a bird. Bennett crawls over to the yellow car. I think he's going to take it away, and that Avery will cry, and that I'll have to intervene. But no. Bennett gets it and brings it to Avery, all without missing a beat.

I have an idea. I take the yellow car and hide it underneath the corner of a baby blanket, a little test. I want to see if Avery will find the toy, or forget about it once it's out of sight. It's one of the concepts on the E-LAP called object permanence. For a moment, Avery looks away from me, out the window to the rain trailing down the windowpane. I think it's too hard for him, and prepare to give in and return the toy. Avery shifts his weight, rolls back onto his tummy, stretches to his full ski jumper and lifts the blanket to get to the car.

I can't believe what's happened. I'm so overjoyed that I swoop him up in my arms and spin around, hooray! I put on a Nina Simone CD, *Little Girl Blue*, "My Baby Just Cares for Me." I pick up both babies, one in each arm, and we dance and sway in celebration. After a while, I can feel Bennett's body grow heavy with sleep; I gently put him in the swing to rest. Then I bring Avery close, inhaling the smell of him, soap and lavender baby lotion and sweet, milky breath. I can feel his heart beating against my own, I can feel his little quick breaths against my neck. Holding him soothes me, and my worry trails away, like raindrops down the windowpane. The song ends, and I keep dancing until

I can feel him breathing deeply, and slowly. He is asleep. I gently lay him in the Pack 'n Play, my baby who just cares for me.

On the kitchen counter is a small white microwave, on top of which is command central. It's not much to look at unless you know my methods—it's where I put all my "important papers." I take out the stack of Wendy's photocopies, my homework for the week. The copies are made from *Gross Motor Skills in Children with Down Syndrome: A Guide for Parents and Professionals.*

The notes begin with chapter three, called "Stage 3: Pivoting, Sitting, and Preparation for Standing," and I feel a little stab of regret over the missing first two chapters—maybe Avery would be crawling already if we'd started therapy sooner. I push the feeling aside and begin reading the activity guidelines, which are simple and straightforward. Each section includes black-and-white photos of very cute babies doing the activities, and I'm particularly taken in by them. And I notice a section on "temperament," which describes two types of learners: motor-driven children, who like the activity of going from one position to another, and observers, who may resist new movements until they become familiar with them. *Aha,* I think. *Here is one of my questions about Avery, answered.* He's an observer.

"Stage 4: Crawling, Quadruped, Climbing, Moving in and out of Sitting, Pulling to Stand, and Standing" is the next assignment for me and Avery. The very first guideline reads, "Do not expect your child to develop the skills of this stage in a particular order." In this chapter, the children in the photos are many ages—some are babies, some look to be two- and three-year-olds. I remember the chart of developmental milestones adjusted for children with Down syndrome in Stray-Gundersen's *Babies with Down Syndrome* and notice the absence of age ranges here. I like it. It feels freeing to let go of the charts and boxes and graphs.

It feels so good, in fact, that even though I've reached the end of my homework, I wish I had more. I want to read ahead, to get the big picture. I want the map of how we will get to the point of Avery walking, from where we are, at the ski jumper. I think back to the stacks of baby books I read when I was a new mom to Carter: *Touchpoints*, *The Womanly Art of Breastfeeding*, *How to Raise Children at Home in Your Spare Time*, *A Parent's Guide to Safety*, *Babyhood*, *The Baby Book: Everything You Need to Know About Your Baby from Birth to Age Two*, all in the first month. My feelings are familiar, and my motives are similar. I want to feel like I understand Avery so that I can support him, and be a good mother to him, as he grows. I want to figure out my son.

Avery and I make the trek down the long corridor of the hospital's physical therapy wing, past the empty reception desk. The walls are beige; the carpet is gray; the artwork is prints of wildlife and Western landscapes. Here, the paintings are all hung low, for people in wheelchairs, and children. The first room we pass on the left looks like a gym, filled with exercise equipment and free weights and floor mats. Wendy's room is the last one at the end of the hall.

Inside, a window faces a brick wall. Below the window, in one corner of the room, is a child-size trampoline. Across from that, there's a wall covered with Peg-Board, where various physical therapy contraptions hang, including a scooter and a swing. More equipment is lined up neatly on the floor below the Peg-Board: a giant purple Tupperware, a royal blue bouncy ball, a royal blue barrel made of rigid foam. Against a third wall is a chair. The room is lit by an overhead fluorescent light.

I sit in the chair and first take off my coat, then my shoes. Next, I unbuckle Avery from the baby carrier and take off his coat, shoes, and socks. He seems to do better with bare feet. While I'm getting us ready, Wendy asks how our week has been. I like that she encourages me to ask questions. She makes me feel as if I were a good mom to Avery.

"I was wondering if we should be doing Avery's therapy a set number of times each day, like exercises?" I ask.

"No," she says. "It should be a part of everyday life. It should feel like play to him. Try to work on these motions as many times as you can, as often as you can, in the normal course of the day. Some days will be better than others—do what you can." She's a mom of two small children and understands, without my having to explain, what our days at home are like.

"What about pain?" I ask. "He seemed really worn-out, last time. Are his muscles hurting? Should I give him ibuprofen?"

"He might be tired, but a nap should take care of it. You don't need to give him anything for pain relief. Muscles don't experience pain from exercise until children are older."

I hesitate, trying to decide if I should ask about the missing two chapters, about the work we might have done, if we'd begun sooner. I can't change the past, I decide, so I let it go.

We begin the bouncy ball work, me doing most of it as Wendy watches. I can already feel that Avery is stronger, can see that he's more in control. He seems pleased with himself, too. I think he likes being able to manage his body.

"I want to try something else," Wendy says. "It's a bit more difficult, but kids don't develop in a straight line. Development is more like in circles, with areas of overlap."

She pulls out a giant purple Tupperware. The lid pops off and inside are hundreds of multicolored balls. She puts Avery in the ball pit. His frowny face comes out immediately. He stretches his arms out, reaching for me to pick him up, and when I don't, he begins crying.

Wendy lifts him up, sits him on the ground, and rolls the blue foam barrel in front of him. I guess she means to entice him to crawl through it. *Good luck,* I think. I've tried this all before, or some variation of it, a hundred times at home.

But no, she positions herself at one end of the barrel, Avery at the other. She's setting up a game, looking at him through the circular opening and encouraging him to do the same. Left, right, outside, inside, "Peek-a-boo!"

Avery laughs.

She does it again. Left, right, outside, inside, "Peek-a-boo!" Avery begins copying her.

Left, right, "Peek-a-boo!"

Avery is playing, too.

Left, right, "Peek-a-boo!"

Avery takes the lead. Left, right, peek!

They both go fast now. Left, right, peek!

And finally, Avery makes his move: Left, *left,* peek!

He catches her off guard; Wendy goes the wrong way. Laugh laugh laugh. He's smiling, proud of himself for his joke. Laugh laugh laugh.

Wendy's eyes grow big, and she laughs, too. "You stinker," she says. "You faked me out!"

Brittney comes to the house for her regular visit. Avery is still doing the ski jumper instead of crawling, and I show her what Wendy and I are working on with the bouncy ball. Brittney gives me photocopies from a book about fine motor skills; Avery's most recent E-LAP shows no delay in this area, but if we want, we can schedule time with an occupational therapist just to be safe. Or, I could do things at home, from the book.

Part of her job, Brittney tells me, is to keep the global view of Avery's development in mind: the big picture. For that reason, she says, she's brought us something. She seems proud, and also a little bit shy, which immediately makes me curious.

I sit on the floor with Avery in my lap, and we wait as she fetches her giant black bag, the one that usually holds binders and papers and stray toys. She returns and pulls the mysterious something from her giant bag. I feel a bit like when Carter shows me his most recent picture for approval, and it takes a minute for my mind to register what I'm seeing.

A coffee can.

A Kirkland decaf can with the label mostly removed and a slot cut in its green plastic lid. She hands it to me, nodding, and says, "Look inside!"

I peel off the lid to reveal an assortment of pink and green plastic coins, and what look like broken plastic clothespins. I don't know what to say.

"For his pincer grasp," she says.

For a moment, I'm confused. Avery can't even crawl. Why are we worrying about his *pincer grasp*?

Avery leans out from my lap, straining toward the coffee can. It's shiny, and the coins and pulled-apart clothespins make a nice rattling sound.

He sits up taller, trying to reach it. I pull it close enough to us that he can get it on his own. He does. Brittney sits across from us.

"I was trying to think of things that would force him to use his index finger and his thumb, together. But I didn't want it to be anything he could choke on. I thought of the coins, but then I realized that might be too easy for him. He could use his palmar grasp with those. Then it came to me: the clothespins!"

Avery begins shaking the can. I can feel that he's using his trunk muscles to control his body as he moves the weight in his hands.

She helps Avery dump out the clothespins and the coins in a pile next to the can, and she replaces the lid. Bennett joins us, and he and Avery take turns putting things through the slot in the lid. After each addition, there is a satisfying *plink*.

Both boys are taking turns, and each boy is using a pincer grasp, particularly with the clothespins. Brittney is proud. Bennett is proud; Avery is proud, too.

I'm humbled.

No one can take away Avery's Down syndrome. Brittney can't give me a cure, or even know all the answers. What she can give me is her concern, her attention. She'd been thinking about us, worrying about Avery's pincer grasp, and so she created a toy to help him. All that good energy. All that care, all that love. This is what she's giving us, a wellspring of support that has most recently manifested itself in the form of a recycled coffee can. It took me a while to see it for what it is.

My homework from Brittney is *Fine Motor Skills for Children with Down Syndrome: A Guide for Parents and Professionals.* The first chapter is called "Introduction: A Parent's Perspective," which tells the story of the author, Maryanne Bruni, and her experiences as an occupational therapist and a mother of a daughter with Down syndrome. I flip through the book and notice more cute photos. There are sections called "Grandma's and Grandpa's List," which are chapter-appropriate lists of toys and equipment that families might appreciate receiving from a grandparent. There's a section on preprinting and printing readiness, which I wish I'd had for Carter. And Bruni takes the idea of letting go of "stages of development" one step further: she writes about "components of development" instead, because at any stage, she feels, there are several components developing at once. I couldn't agree more; I decide that maybe I'll want to have my own copy of this book, too, my wish list slowly growing.

Seventeen years ago, the man and his wife who built our house fenced off a little rectangle below the porch and planted perennials. Now, like a true teenager, the garden has gone wild with a heady independence. The giant yellow forsythia blooms first in a massive, arcing spray. The white lilac tree is next—in the moonlight, the clusters of tiny blooms shine like pearls. There are deep purple lilacs, pink and purple columbine, grape hyacinth, everything overgrown and out of control. When the peonies burst open, the scent is so strong, even the bees get drunk. And though it's barely the end of March, the temperature has been in the fifties and I can't wait any longer. I need to get my hands in the dirt and smell its richness. I want to feel the crumbling of freshly turned soil between my fingers and beneath my nails.

It's a sunny day, so I bundle up everyone and strap the babies into the stroller and we all go down the hill to the patch of lawn and the garden gate. I settle the babies on a quilt on the grass and leave them with Carter, playing. I begin loosening the soil around the stumps of peonies. I notice a yellowish glow to the forsythia branches that tells me the flowers are nearly ready to bloom. I'm digging, happy. I uncover a barrette with three sparkly blue stars on it, probably from one of the two Graces Carter sometimes plays with. I brush the barrette off and put it in my hair so I won't lose it before I can return it to its rightful little-girl owner.

I look over at the babies. Bennett has rolled over and is trying to eat grass. Avery is pumping his fist, open, closed, open, closed. The air smells sweet and I can feel life humming all around me.

"What are you thinking about?" I yell to Carter.

"My candy collection," he yells back. Carter has saved every piece of candy he's ever gotten in a large white box that he keeps on the top shelf of the bookcase. From time to time he takes it down and admires the individually wrapped Fireballs, the assortment of Dum Dums, the Smarties and Jolly Ranchers and Sugar Babies. He watches over the candy, arranging it in the box just so, and when he's done, he returns it to its high shelf amidst the novels and anthologies of poems.

"What are you thinking about?" Carter asks me.

"My garden," I answer, envisioning the peonies and the forsythia, the daisies and the buttercups, the raised beds where I grow vegetables, and as I do, I realize my son and I are thinking about essentially the same thing—abundance.

Carter begins playing with a ball, I keep digging, and the next thing I know Avery is peering at me from the foot of the garden bed. I'm surprised, then confused. It's much too far for him to have traveled on his own.

"How did Avery get here?" I ask Carter.

"Taxi ride, Mommy," he says.

"What?"

"I gave Avery a taxi ride," he says.

My first thought is, *How does he know about taxis?* My second thought: *That's so sweet!* Any my third: *I wonder if this is why Avery isn't crawling yet.*

"Carter, honey, do you give Avery taxi rides very often?"

"Sure, Mommy. He can't get around on his own," he says. "Devin does it, too, and Shaver, and sometimes Russell. We all help him."

"Oh, I see," I answer, wondering what to make of this thoughtful, potentially harmful new development. "I love how you are so kind to your brothers," I begin. "But let's try a new thing. Let me show you how we can help Avery learn to crawl on his own so we don't need to give him taxi rides anymore. When we get up to the house, you can help me do Avery's exercises with him. And when we go to Avery's class, maybe you can come, too, and meet Wendy. She's a special teacher who knows about bodies and muscles and how they work. She can help both of us learn the best ways to help Avery."

I look over at him to see if he's listening. He's digging in the dirt with my hand trowel, looking for worms. I repeat myself, to be sure he understands: "Sometimes helping someone is not doing it for them, but teaching them how to do it themselves."

And then: "No more taxi rides, unless it's an emergency."

When Tom gets home, I leave the kids with him and drive to my new favorite grocery store with a different bakery section. In the parking lot, pushing around stray shopping carts, is a big pigeon-toed Avery-man. He's trying very hard, working up a sweat as he wrangles the carts into order. I think I should help him; or maybe I shouldn't. I don't know which is best.

I want to speak with him, engage him, make up for all the other times I passed by people with learning differences or physical differences and ignored them. I want to know about his life: Where does he live? Who are his friends? His family—where do they live? Who is his mother? Even as I form these questions, I recognize I have no right to ask them. Seeing this man means I see him in totality—he's not here to help me feel better. He's busy working, and taking time to assuage my guilt could get him fired. That's the last thing I want to do. I nod "hello" in what I hope is a friendly and supportive way, and I move on.

The spring plant selection is set up in front of the store. An elderly man holds a tomato plant, inspecting it, turning it carefully, gingerly, as if his making the right choice is a matter of tremendous consequence. Farther down, a skinny woman with a long ponytail selects a bright orange marigold. She puts it back, and instead reaches for a yellow one. The bright pompon of the flower reminds me of an egg yolk, two egg yolks, twins. My babies.

I'm struck by the moment. That life goes on. That Avery has Down syndrome, that everything moves forward with such beauty and tenderness and sincerity. I touch something in my hair and realize it's the sparkly barrette I'd found in the garden. Three stars, three sons, shining.

# 12

❧

# More, More

Molly is a woman in her late twenties with shoulder-length brown hair and large green eyes. Her office, in the same part of the hospital as Wendy's, is the size of a closet. Me, Molly, Avery, and Avery's baby carrier barely fit. I put the baby carrier outside in the hall.

To Avery, speech therapy is party time. Molly feeds him chocolate pudding, showing me how to keep the baby spoon flat and even, which encourages him to use the muscles around his mouth, as opposed to my method, which is to scrape the food off the spoon using his gums. She shows him how to sip juice from a plastic teddy bear with a clear straw on top, while I shrink into the background thinking, *He's only a baby—he still needs a bottle!* Avery proves me wrong, sipping away like an old pro; he's very proud of himself, plus he likes the juice.

When Molly speaks, she uses a loud, clear voice, and if Avery isn't looking at her, she positions herself so that she's in his line of sight. She does these things easily, as if it were second nature. When I try to do them, I feel silly, like I'm talking to an eighty-year-old man instead of a nine-month-old baby.

She shows me a Nuk tool, which looks like a toothbrush with plastic knobs on the end, and explains that it's good for oral-motor stimulation. "Or you could use any toothbrush, too," she says, "especially the *motorized ones that make funny noises when we stick them in our mouths.*" As she says this last part, she moves around so her face is right in Avery's face, and she's speaking only to him. He smiles his big smile, flirting a little bit.

The Speech Therapy Party Time list goes on: curly straws and bendy straws and straws with paper sleeves on them. Harmonicas and kazoos and recorders and whistles and party horns with paper streamers. A pink plastic elephant that holds bubble solution and a shiny silver pinwheel and a whirligig in the shape of a puppy. Treats of course, more chocolate pudding and juice from the teddy bear. "Never a sippy cup," Molly reminds me. *"We never, ever drink from a sippy cup because it doesn't work the muscles of our mouths,"* she says slowly and clearly to Avery.

I'm familiar with the ideas behind the toys after watching Libby Kumin in *The First 18 Months* (the DVD Brittney loaned us). In order to have clear speech, Avery needs several skills. He needs to be able to hold and release air from his lungs in a sustainable and modulated way, hence the horns and other blowing-type activities. He needs to be able to control the muscles in his face and around his mouth, which the straw work and the oral-motor stimulation help him practice. And he needs to learn that people communicate with each other by combining these skills to produce sounds that have meaning, ideas that are enforced by Molly's animated tones and exaggerated speech patterns. The more I am around her, the more comfortable I become speaking to Avery this way, too.

She has books for me to read: *Early Communication Skills* and *The New Language of Toys.* She loans them to me with the condition that I promise to *"Give them back to Molly when Mom's all done reading them."*

Molly's books become additions to my wish list. *The New Language of Toys* reinforces Molly's way of speaking to Avery and gives me suggestions for more ways of incorporating it into our lives. Toys can speak to Avery, for example, and I can narrate our lives to him, too, by telling him the story of what I'm doing as I'm doing it. It's the smallest of all the books in my stack, and it focuses mostly on teaching language throughout the day. Like the others, it includes photos of children of all ages, working at the activities described in the chapters. And again, I'm drawn to the images of the kids—playing, smiling, laughing, and learning.

*Early Communication Skills for Children with Down Syndrome: A Guide for Parents and Professionals* includes material similar to what was presented in the DVD Brittney shared with us, but in much greater detail. The book begins with several points to remember: Communication is holistic, meaning that it's more than the sum of its parts. Communication gains meaning through relationship—what is said, for example, is influenced by how it is said. Communication may be intentional or unintentional; and it includes verbal as well as nonverbal messages.

Language can be thought of as an arbitrary, shared code that uses symbols to represent real objects and events. There are rules about how we use the code, which are learned through social interaction. Language is intentional and purposeful; it may include gestures, signs, pictures, and/or speech.

Speech is defined as a verbal language that uses the same systems in the body that are used for breathing, swallowing, and eating. Creating speech involves muscle programming, muscle movement, and muscle coordination.

Learning about what I'd always called "talking" in these new terms is exciting, and fascinating. I took so much of this for granted with Carter. Language as a code; deciphering verbal and nonverbal clues; words as just one of the many means of communication—it feels as if my mind and heart are expanding. I, too, am learning a new way: the way of Avery, and other children like him.

It's snowing again, a late spring storm of big wet flakes that melt as soon as they touch the bare window boxes or the wooden planks of the porch. Bennett follows me around from room to room, working on his stiff-legged gait. He says, "Mama-mama-mama," and Avery says it, too, copying him, "Mmm-mmm-mmm." Carter notices and says, "The babies call you Mama, Mommy. Isn't that funny?"

There are no therapy appointments today, no trips to doctors or to town for groceries. On days like this, home with my children, it's easy. We watch VHS tapes, we dance, we play. We take naps. We build blanket forts and then bake cookies and eat them in the blanket forts. On days at home, I forget there's any trouble here at all.

One of the VHS tapes we have to watch is called *Signing Time!*, a sign language video for children. Part of Avery's speech therapy is learning sign language, to help reinforce the concept that people can ask for things, and communicate with each other through words and, until he's able to say words, gestures.

The *Signing Time!* tape begins with a woman with long brown hair, parted in the middle, wearing a red shirt. She's about my age, and to me she looks like a mom—strong hands with short nails that might have washed a lot of little bodies and wiped many dirty faces; no necklaces or earrings that small hands could pull; a wash-and-wear shirt. And it's more than her appearance; it's a quiet confidence that comes from having been up all night, holding a sick baby or rocking a teething infant, and knowing that you could do it again the next night, and the next, if you had to.

She's singing a song with the lyrics, "It's signing time with Alex and Leah / It's signing time with Alex and Leah / Come and play." As she sings, her hands make the signs for the words to the song. When the music ends, the word "eat" appears onscreen, and a woman's voice reads it aloud. The woman in the red shirt reappears and demonstrates the sign for *eat*, which is a hand to the mouth, as if you were eating. As she makes the sign, she repeats the word loudly and clearly, "Eat. Eat. Eat."

The scene changes to a series of shots of babies, toddlers, and children making the sign, too, and a voice-over of a young girl saying, "This is the sign for *eat*." Interspersed throughout the demonstrations are quick images of various children playing, or swinging, or eating, and also signing. Babies, toddlers, kids—all signing. Mothers, fathers, grandparents—everyone signs. The visual message is strong and appealing to me: using sign language is a natural part of everyday life, something families and children do together.

Many of the signs look just as you might think they would: *More* is touching your fingers together twice, more-more. *Thirsty* is a finger tracing a line down the throat. *Sleepy* is a hand over the face, closing the eyes. *No* is the thumb and the index finger pinching shut. *Dog* (pat your thigh), *cat* (pinch your hands near your nose like whiskers), *fish* (wiggle a flat hand like a fish gliding through the water). I put Avery in my lap and take his hands in mine and together we practice, hand over hand. When we accomplish whatever sign we are working on, he smiles and laughs; I can't tell if he understands what we're doing, or if he simply likes my enthusiasm at his success.

Later in the afternoon, the snow changes to rain. Carter colors at the dining room table. Bennett walks from couch to chair to chair in a little line that I've set up for him; it looks like an abandoned game of musical chairs. And Avery plays on the floor near the couch, beneath the Gymini. A few feet away, the rain hits the window, *pat pat pat.* I can hear raindrops on the roof. I'm thinking about my garden, and how good the rain is for it. When I look back to the window, Avery's beneath it, straining to pull up to the windowsill.

I can't believe what I see. *How did he get there?* My excitement builds—it almost hurts to hope.

"Carter, did you move Avery?" I ask.

"No, Mommy. I'm doing crayons. It's a house," he says.

I look from the Gymini to the window, trying to calculate all the possibilities. Bennett is too far away, Tom is down in the office, and Carter didn't help him. That only leaves one scenario: Avery did it. Avery did it, himself! At first, I'm so overjoyed I'm speechless. Then, for a quick moment, I think, *I'm with him all the time, and I missed it! I can't believe I missed it!*

*"Do you want to stand, Avery?"* I say and go to him, and help him stand up to the window like Wendy showed me, cueing his muscles and letting him do the work. He's happy, and laughing. I laugh, too, and kiss the top of his head and rub his back, saying, *"Who's standing? Who's standing and looking out the window? Is it raining? Look at the rain!"*

Molly has arranged a speech therapy play group at the local nursing home. Avery and I are the first to reach the locked front door, where we wait to be buzzed in. I wave to the little camera at the entrance, lift up the baby carrier with Avery inside. The door clicks, I pull it open, and I can hear Molly's cheerful voice saying, *"Here we are, down the hall in the activity room."*

An old brown-and-orange plaid couch and matching love seat are arranged in front of an entertainment center that holds a television, a VHS player, and a stereo. To the left is a brown plastic accordion wall that has been pulled shut, to close off the other half of the room. Molly has laid a quilt on top of the thin gray carpet. On it are a barnyard set and the corresponding animals.

Molly's supervisor is visiting today and I recall Molly telling me that the woman has a brother with Down syndrome. We introduce ourselves, and I notice a smear of black mascara underneath her right eye. I become distracted by this, wondering if I should say something or ignore it. Is it better to ignore it? But sometime today, she'll notice it, and then she'll think back, *Who did I talk to?* And she'll wonder if I knew, and maybe feel like I should have mentioned it. She's saying something; I should be paying attention. She's saying something about Avery.

"And so that's why I think it shouldn't even be questioned; I think all children with Down syndrome should have their tonsils and adenoids taken out."

She's wearing a business suit and she has long red nails. I can't imagine that she has children. *I am such a judgmental person,* I think, realizing that I split the whole world into two groups: moms and not-moms.

"Okay, sure, tonsils and adenoids out, I understand," I say. I file this away in my mind, but I hope it doesn't come to that; I don't want to go back to the hospital, ever.

I put Avery on the quilt, and he ski jumps and wriggles and squirms his way off of it, heading straight for the entertainment center. He's got his eye on the stereo, and when he gets there he pulls himself up to look at it. I'm right behind him, in case he falls, or touches something he shouldn't.

Molly claps and says to me, "Wow! This is new, isn't it?"

I grin. Both she and her supervisor say in unison, *"Way to go, Avery!"*

Another woman arrives, a mom with a baby in a carrier. She looks young and bewildered. An old man materializes in the doorway behind her, and peers around at us, confused. Behind him, a blond woman takes his arm and guides him away. The young mom gets a fearful look in her eyes, as if she's trying to decide whether to join us or bolt. I smile at her, unsure what else to do. Her baby is small, about the size of a three-month-old. I think he's a boy; I see that he has a rashy face from where a cannula might have been. She smiles back at me, then looks at Avery.

"Yours?" she asks.

I nod. She sets the baby carrier down facing her and sinks into the plaid couch. I recognize this move: turning the baby into you means no one can see, which means fewer questions. I can tell she wants to ask me more but doesn't know how. She's curious, maybe even in a good, kind way. She's looking to me for an explanation; of Avery, of me and my life, which is part of being Avery's mom that I hadn't expected. She wants to know how it feels to be Avery's mom.

There were so many times in the past when I wanted to tell my story but didn't. So many things I wanted to say but couldn't. Here, I have an audience. Now, I am ready. I begin. I start slowly, telling about the twins, the surprise. I tell the part about the NICU, and how scared I was. Tears come into my eyes; talking about it is going to be harder than I thought.

"I was in the NICU, too," she says. "Who was your doctor?"

I tell her about Doc Hollywood, and the lemon sherbet pediatrician, and the nurses I remember. She doesn't recognize any of the names, but it doesn't matter. She begins telling her story, which includes preeclampsia, a micropreemie, and three months in the NICU.

I remember Owen, the twenty-seven-weeks baby who had an isolette next to the twins. I look at the young mother more closely, to see if she resembles the woman I met that night in the hospital. But no, it's not her. It doesn't matter; I feel as if I know her, anyway. She's my sister in this experience; I empathize, and admire her for being in the NICU for that long.

"I don't know how you managed it," I say.

"I don't know, either," she says, eyes welling with tears, and I can see that I've said the wrong thing. I calculate the dates; she must have just gotten home.

"It's so good to be home," I say quietly. "That's all I care about. That we're home, and we're together. We have the rest of our lives to sort all the other stuff out," I add, which feels true, in an oversimplified way.

The old man reappears at the doorway. He's wearing a flannel robe and has a shock of white hair. He seems gentle and harmless. He wants to see the babies. I take Avery in my arms and bring him to the man. I say, "This is Avery." He has a haze to his pale blue eyes and I wonder if he can understand me, if he can even see. I wonder who his people are, how he got here; we all have a story, and I wonder what his might be.

I think back to Emily Perl Kingsley's "Welcome to Holland" essay, and the need for an easy way to explain what it feels like to be Avery's mom. I can't put my finger on it. Maybe there isn't an easy way to explain it. Or maybe there is: It feels just like you think it'd feel. It feels like being a mother.

The old man's aide comes to fetch him, and as she turns him away, he says, "You have a beautiful son."

I nod, and lift Avery's tiny, pudgy hand to wave bye-bye.

The piano, and my notes of hope. The click of the bedroom door, which Avery wakes to instantly. The telephone ringing. The way he turns when I call his name, even at a whisper. These are the things that give me confidence that Avery can hear.

Since our disastrous hearing exam in the hospital chapel, I've done some research, and Molly has given me the name of a different audiologist, a woman who is also a speech therapist and works with children. I've made an appointment with her in Missoula to have Avery retested. While we're there, we'll also have his eyes checked by a pediatric ophthalmologist with offices in the same building. I prefer to batch the doctor appointments together, so I can get them done as quickly and painlessly as possible. I also schedule the first appointment of the day whenever I can, so I have a better chance of spending less time in the waiting room. And I bring snacks and say thank you a lot, which seems to help everyone, me especially.

Now that Avery's older, there are more ways to test his hearing. The goal is to determine which sounds Avery can hear; the softest noise he can hear 50 percent of the time is called a threshold. There are two ways of determining a threshold: behavioral testing, which relies on Avery's responses to evaluate his level of hearing, and objective testing, which uses machines to take measurements.

Behavioral tests include Visual Reinforcement Audiometry (VRA), a method used with children five months to two years old. The child sits on a parent's lap in a sound booth and is taught to look toward (orient to) a sound coming through a loudspeaker. When the child looks toward the correct speaker, a lighted moving toy is switched on as a reward.

Conditioned Play Audiometry (CPA) is a second form of behavioral test used with children slightly older than Avery, two- to five-year-olds. In CPA, each time a sound is heard, the child is encouraged to perform an activity, such as putting a block in a bucket, or a peg in a Peg-Board. When the child does these things, the reward is the lighted moving toy, and also praise from the tester and the parent.

The third type of behavioral test is called Conventional Audiometry (CA), which is useful for children age five years and older. In CA, a child is asked to raise his hand when he hears a tone, and repeat sounds and words as instructed. The reward is praise, from the parent and the tester.

Objective testing methods don't require a child's participation, which makes them popular choices for small children and even babies. Otoacoustic Emissions (OAE) is an objective test in which sounds are presented to a child through a small rubber probe that measures otoacoustic emission, which is generated by hair cells in the inner ear. This is the test Avery and I abandoned previously, leaving the hospital chapel in tears.

Auditory Brainstem Response (ABR) is another kind of objective testing that requires natural sleep or sedation. Small electrodes are taped to the child's head, sounds are played, and the response of the hearing nerve and auditory pathway at the base of the brain are measured. ABR testing is sometimes referred to as Auditory Brainstem Evoked Response testing (ABER), or

Brainstem Auditory Evoked Response testing (BAER). It's the test that I refused for Avery, because of the sedation.

The third type of objective testing is called a Tympanometry/Impedance Test, which measures the function of the middle ear system—the eardrum, the middle ear bones, and the eustachian tube. When a loud sound is presented to a healthy ear, the eardrum will contract in an acoustic reflex. To complete a tympanogram, a probe is placed in the ear; then a vacuum-tight seal is created. The air pressure in the ear canal is changed, and the movement of the eardrum is measured and recorded.

The receptionist looks bored and is eating M&Ms from a glass bowl. She has sunglasses perched on top of her head, as if she's just popped inside for a moment. Avery and I pick up the forms to fill out, and again, there's no place to put "Down syndrome." I write it across the top and add stars to it, as before. The receptionist takes the clipboard from me and motions for us to sit and wait.

In the room with us is a woman dressed entirely in pink—pink heels, pink nylons, pink sweater. Briefly, I wonder why she's here. *She's probably thinking the same thing about us*, I decide. Across from her is a display of hearing aid batteries, and next to that, a magazine rack. I set Avery's baby carrier down next to me and thumb through the selection: *New Yorker, Rolling Stone, Nickelodeon.* A book about a mouse called *Oliver Gets Hearing Aids.* Before I can make a choice, the new audiologist comes out and introduces herself.

"Hi, I'm Eve," she says. She has blond hair, blue eyes, and pale skin. She's wearing jeans and a maroon fleece Columbia vest. Two diamond studs twinkle in her ears.

She shows us to the test booth, and positions me in a chair with Avery on my lap. Then she closes the door and disappears. Her voice comes from a speaker on the right: "Avery, Avery,

Avery." Avery turns to it, and a Minnie Mouse doll flashes red, red, red. She nods at me through the little plastic window and then gives me a thumbs-up. We go again, this time a sound from the left speaker: "Avery, Avery, Avery." He turns to the left; more lights go off, this time blue. The test continues, each sound growing softer and softer, until I can't even hear it any longer. I see the thumbs-up again, and the booth's door opens.

"He did great!" she says. "I want to try something else," she adds, and hands me a wooden board with pictures painted on it, a dog and a cat and a cow. "I'll say the words, and let's see if he repeats them," she explains.

"He's not really talking yet," I say, "but we're learning sign language."

"He can sign, then, or point. Let's try it," she says.

The door closes as she disappears and soon I hear, "Dog, dog, dog." Avery squirms in my lap. I hear it again, "Dog, dog, dog."

Avery is trying to lick the board. I hear, "You can help him with the sign, hand over hand."

I take Avery's hand and pat it on his thigh, saying, "Dog, dog, dog." Then I take his finger and point to the picture of the dog.

Next I hear, "Cat, cat, cat." Avery squirms again, and out comes the frowny face. I look toward the little window, but I can't see anyone. I try to bring Avery's fingers to his nose to make the whiskery sign for kitty, but he resists me, arching his back and trying to twist away.

The door to the booth opens and Eve comes in. "I think we're done with the booth," she says. "Just wait here a minute." She disappears again, this time leaving the door open.

In a moment, the Minnie Mouse flashes red, blue, red, blue, and a burst of music and the sound of a crowd cheering come over the speakers. *"Good job, Avery. Hooray for Avery!"* Avery likes this, and begins clapping.

Eve reappears in the doorway. "I like to end on a positive

note. It makes the kids happy to come back and get tested again. We want to keep it a good experience."

She tells me to fit him back into his car seat, and we have one more thing to try. I buckle him in, and she takes out what looks like a long thin stick attached to a wire, which connects to a little box. She seems to want to put the stick in his ear. I'm nervous; since the OAE, Avery has been extremely touchy about his ears. She proceeds quickly, placing a probe in each of Avery's ears before I can explain how impossible it will be. Then she's gone again, and back. In her hand is a curled paper that looks like a printout from an ATM.

"This is the most beautiful tympanogram I've ever seen," she says, smiling.

I look at her, stunned. "Really?" I manage.

"Yes, really. I wish all kids had such clear ear canals." She smiles at me again, diamonds twinkling, kindness in her voice. I see in her a woman who must know what it's like to be on the receiving end of bad news. She's a woman who knows how to celebrate the good news, too.

"Thank you," I say. "Thank you so much." I'm so grateful. Giddy with relief. High with happiness. And ready to face the ophthalmologist. I have horrible vision myself, but Tom has the eyes of an eagle. Why not hope? Hope for the best.

Avery and I make our way farther into the maze of cubicles and reception rooms. It's nearing lunchtime and most of the offices are quiet, empty. I find the correct receptionist and fill out more forms. Again, I have to write "Down syndrome" across the top, adding my stars, tra-la! This time, we are ushered straight into the exam room.

The doctor introduces himself and explains that he's going to check Avery for nearsightedness, farsightedness, astigmatism, eye movement ability, proper eye alignment, reaction to changes in light and darkness, and any general eye health problems. He is about my age, and wears a sport coat and tie. He seems friendly and professional; I detect no ill will toward Avery.

The eye exam will consist of an assessment of ocular alignment ("Are the eyes straight and do they work together?" he explains), an assessment of ocular movement ("Do the eyes move normally?" he says), an estimate of visual acuity, and an assessment of the need for glasses.

"What are your plans for the rest of the day?" he asks.

"Um, we'll be driving home," I answer.

"Good. Then I'd like to recommend a dilated eye exam, which will allow me to look at Avery's retina. The drops take a while to wear off, is why I ask."

He motions for me to sit in an exam chair with Avery on my lap; he pulls out a wheeled, swiveling stool for himself, then straps what looks like a tiny rock climber's light on his head. He leans in to Avery, then leans out, focusing all the while on Avery's eyes. "Has he ever had excessive tearing, swelling, or crusting?" he asks, leaning in again.

"No," I say. He leans out.

"Have you noticed him squinting, or rubbing his eyes?" he asks, flipping up the light and turning it on.

"Only when he's tired," I say. "He rubs his eyes when he's ready to go to sleep."

He turns the light off and flips it down, then wheels himself behind us and slowly around us, right to left, peering at Avery as he rolls around our chair.

He produces a stuffed teddy bear and holds it up, slowly moving it to the left, then the right, all the while watching Avery's eyes. He removes the headband.

"I'm going to ask you to hold his head steady while I look into his eyes with the ophthalmoscope. What this test does is show any abnormalities in the back of the eye, or cataracts, or other clouding of the eye lens."

I cup my fist under Avery's chin and the doctor wheels in about a foot away from us, shining what looks like a radar gun toward each of Avery's eyes. The red reflex in each eye is symmetrical, which is good, he explains. Then he asks me to let go of Avery's chin; he rolls over to a dimmer switch on the wall and lowers the lights. From a panel in the wall about three feet away, a glowing stuffed monkey appears, then disappears. Avery is delighted. A second panel opens farther from us; it's a lit-up cow. Avery claps. A third panel opens, farther still. A frog; Avery claps again.

"Good and good," the doctor says, turning up the lights. "One last thing. I'm going to put these drops in his eyes, and they will take about thirty minutes to work. You can wait here and I'll be back shortly."

He holds Avery's head steady, squeezes one drop into each of his eyes, points to a box of toys in the corner, and leaves.

The exam has gone quickly, and I'm not sure what to think. I want to believe that if there were a problem, the doctor would have told me. I want to assume that no news means good news, but I have learned never to assume anything.

I have a bottle in my diaper bag for Avery that I'd been hoping to give him right before we left Missoula, so that he'd sleep on the ride home. I give it to him now, instead. He's been such a good boy, so patient and cooperative. I go to the dimmer switch and turn the lights down a bit, and sit in the exam chair, and hold Avery, rocking and singing to him quietly. He stares up at me with his big blue eyes, the white stars in them twinkling.

When the doctor returns, I've finished feeding Avery his bottle and we've begun playing with a green monster truck from the box in the corner.

"How is Avery doing so far?" I ask.

"He's doing great. His eyes are healthy and working together in a coordinated fashion. This last test will measure if he's near-sighted, farsighted, or has astigmatism."

He indicates that I should retake my position with Avery on my lap in the chair, which I do. He then shines a light into each of Avery's eyes, back and forth.

"What does that do?" I ask, determined to be more proactive.

"The light enters the eye and bounces back," he says. "The way the light behaves as it comes out helps me determine the re-fractive power of the eye."

I cut to the chase. "Does he need glasses?"

"He's a little bit farsighted, but most babies are. He's fine."

He turns off the light, and the exam is over. The last thing he does is reach into a drawer and pull out a tiny pair of blue sunglasses.

"For the dilated pupils," he explains. "They should be back to normal in a few hours. If not, give me a call."

I nod, and thank him.

On our way out, the receptionist asks to take a photocopy of our insurance card. Avery is strapped in his car seat, wearing his sunglasses like a movie star. I set the carrier on the floor, and begin digging around in the diaper bag for my wallet. I look down at Avery and see that he's casually, nonchalantly wriggling his hand through the air, which is the sign for *fish*.

I sign back, *fish,* without giving it much thought, looking for my wallet. I find it in the outside pocket. Avery's still signing, *fish*. I sign back, *fish*. Then I see it, in the corner. A bubbling aquarium with a fish in it. A puffer fish. Taped to the aquarium is a note, "Please do not tap on the glass."

Avery is watching it, making the fish sign. I hand the insur-ance card to the receptionist and pick up the baby carrier and take Avery over to the aquarium so he can better see the fish. I put the carrier in my lap and bend down into his little face wearing the rock-star sunglasses and kiss him on the cheeks, the nose, on his little rosebud mouth, all the while saying, "Fish, Avery, yes! Fish!" and wiggling my hand through the air. My heart is so full of happiness, so full of gratitude, so full of pride that I feel as if I'll burst, just like the puffer fish Avery is watching, and knows now how to name.

Avery and Bennett and Carter and I are with Sarah and her two boys at a local fast-food restaurant that has an indoor play area that we affectionately call Germ Land. But we need a place to go that's out of the rainy day and out of the house and this is it. I've braced myself for the looks, the stares, the questions, because I'm not sure where Germ Land fits on the map of my new life—if it's in the safety zone or the no-fly zone.

Carter and Sarah's boys eat quickly and begin climbing through the brightly colored tunnels that lead to a ball pit. Sarah and I are left with Bennett, who is gnawing on a French fry, and Avery, who is sucking on his fist. Sarah has recently received upsetting news. The baby of a dear friend of hers was diagnosed with trisomy 18, a genetic condition similar to Down syndrome. Sarah wants to know what to say to her friend about her daughter. She's asked me to tell her what I think.

"It's not bad, it's just different," I begin, then falter.

She nods, waiting as I try to explain.

I think about the illusions we live with as parents. How scary everyday life with children can be. How it always seems like there's a wolf at the door; how if you really think about it, there always *is* a wolf at the door. How part of parenting requires that you ignore the wolf; that you proceed as if everything is fine, and hope that it will indeed be fine. Most of the time, it works out that way.

"When you talk with her, don't say, 'I'm sorry,'" I begin again. "No one likes that." I think about what I need as Avery's mom. I need to believe it will be okay. I'm not looking for a happy ending, exactly; I'm not sure if I'd believe it even if one were offered. But I need to know it's bearable.

"These are the things I've begun telling myself," I say. "There are worse things than loving someone and having to care for them. Caring comes naturally, out of that love. And love is both smaller, and bigger, than I'd thought." I realize I'm not making much sense. It's too philosophical. I need to stick to what I know. I look around the play area, searching, trying to collect my thoughts.

I notice a young boy sitting next to us. He's speaking to his mother using sign language. He's signing, *play*, then, *play, please?*

A year ago, I might have wondered what was wrong with the boy. Today, I notice instead that he has many signs, and I see that he's good at them. I wish there was a sign for it, for what I'm trying to tell Sarah.

"It's like this," I try again. "The bee. The bee and the flower. They need each other. You could look at the bee and think, 'There's got to be a better way for you, with all your buzzing around.' And you could look at the flower and think, 'You! You're so dependent! You don't do anything but sit there!' But if you thought those things, you'd be wrong. You'd be missing the point."

Sarah smiles at me, and I can tell I'm still being too theoretical. I try to explain better. "I used to think I wanted my children to grow up to be strong. To be the best, so that they wouldn't need anyone or anything, so that they'd have every choice in life and be able to call all the shots. But that's not right. I don't want them to grow up to be so strong and efficient that they become isolated and alone. I just want my kids to know how to love, and be loved."

Sarah is nodding. She's trying to understand my point. My last try: "You can't have a child, any child, and not be changed by the experience. I'm changed by Avery. And the thing is, I don't want to be changed back." Avery notices the little boy at the next table and waves hello. The boy waves. Avery grins his big grin, proud of himself. The other boy keeps going. *Play*, the boy signs, *play?*

Avery signs, *fish*.

Then Avery makes a new sign, one we've practiced, but I haven't seen him do on his own before. Swinging side to side, hugging himself, back and forth, proud. He's saying, *baby*.

That's the sign I want to use to tell Sarah what it's like being Avery's mom. Big love, big joy. Let go. Hug yourself and swing your body and smile and expect that the world will receive you just as you are, and it will. It will because you make it so, with all your heart and your whole body, smiling, swaying back and forth so fast and pure that the surety of it makes you dizzy.

# 13

## Everybody's Baby but My Own

The sage grouse are drumming. In the spring, the males beat their wings against the ground in a showy dance, trying to attract a mate. The low *thump thump thump* begins slowly and builds on itself, growing louder and faster, and sounds like the start-up of a power lawn mower. It takes me a minute to remember that it's not a suburban Saturday sound, but wings against the forest floor, deep in the woods. It's a sound of life and creation, one that reminds me of the summer I was pregnant.

I'd wanted the chance to fall in love with a baby one more time; I'd wanted to revisit those sleepy, milky, fuzzy newborn days; I'd wanted to feel my body shift and swell, making way for new life. It's true, I'd wanted all these things for myself, but I'd also wanted something for Carter—a sibling. Tom grew up with an older brother; I had a younger sister. All my memories of childhood include her: tree forts made of pillows and blankets; playing Marco Polo in the swimming pool; scraping squished apricots off the hot cement as punishment for sneaking over the back fence and stealing oranges from the neighbor's tree. Dressing the family dog in baby clothes and pushing her around in a doll stroller; playing Wiffle ball in our pajamas in the early evening twilight. My love for my sister was imperfect—her tree fort was always below mine, on a lesser, lower branch; sometimes I'd cheat at Marco Polo by getting out of the pool and going into the house without telling her; I made her clean up the nastiest, mushiest apricots. And yet despite my uneven affections, in her eyes, I could do no wrong.

I'd wanted Carter to have the love of a brother or sister. And as the mother, I'd protect my children from the casual injustices they might inflict upon each other. I'd teach them to say "I love you" and "I'm sorry" and I'd make sure those words were spoken easily and often. I'd be there to smooth hurt feelings and soften unkind words.

These are the choices I made. And now that I have three children, it feels even more important that I nurture their relationships with each other. Like any mother, I hope they grow up to be friends. I hope that when I'm gone, they'll feel my love for them in their love for each other. It's what Tom's parents wish for their sons; it's what my parents wish for my sister and me.

Hope is the note of all our songs.

I pull open the right half of the glass-and-metal double doors of the hospital's physical therapy wing. I hold Avery in my left arm, balancing him on my hip. I jam my foot in front of the door to hold it open, then maneuver us through. Joanne, the receptionist, sees us coming and smiles. She has a little crush on Avery, and the feeling is mutual.

"Here comes my boy!" Joanne says. Avery smiles his biggest smile for her, then buries his face in my neck, laughing.

"Where'd he go?" Joanne asks. Avery pops his head up, still laughing and smiling.

"There he is!" she says.

Again, Avery hides in my neck. Again, there he is!

Joanne interrupts the game to tell me, "It'll just be a minute. Wendy's still with another client." I nod and tell Avery to wave bye-bye, because he's getting heavy on my hip. We make our way to the waiting area, where I sink into a chair. Avery sits at my feet, and begins playing with a fire truck from the toy bin.

Avery sees Wendy before I do; he claps and waves as she walks down the hall toward us. "And how is everyone today?" she asks.

"Fine, good," I say as we follow her back to her room.

Inside, I lower Avery to the floor in front of the chair. I slip off my shoes and put them next to the door. Then I take off Avery's shoes and socks and set them next to mine.

"How has your week been?" Wendy asks.

"Good, mostly. He's still pulling himself up to the window to look out. But I can't get him interested in pulling himself onto the couch, like the book says."

"That's okay," Wendy says. "He'll get it when he's ready. Just keep encouraging him to pull up to the window. He's doing great!"

She disappears into the closet, then reappears with two of Avery's favorite toys: a ball with a bell inside, and a wooden kitty with whiskers. She wiggles the toys and says, "Look what I found!" so that Avery is sure to notice. Then she puts them on the child-size trampoline in the corner, below the window.

Avery takes the bait. As he crawls over to the tramp, Wendy pushes the toys farther back, so they are just out of reach. Avery pulls himself up onto the tramp, so he's standing. Then he leans out, stretching toward the kitty. Wendy is right behind him, ready to support him if he loses his balance. She touches his right leg, helping it bend, lifting it up. Avery responds; he's half on, half off. She touches his other leg, lifting it up, too. Now he scoots across the trampoline and grabs the kitty, happy and proud.

"*Good job, Avery!*" she says. Avery nods, then waits; when we forget to clap for him, he reminds us. Clap, clap, clap. We clap, too. Wendy lets Avery play with the kitty for a bit, then picks him up and moves him back across the room, and the whole process repeats itself, for as long as Avery is willing. When he tires, we stop. Wendy brings over the bell ball, and we practice rolling it back and forth, until our half hour is nearly up.

"Bennett can run now; some days, Avery won't even crawl," I tell Wendy. "It feels as if we're moving so slowly, some days in circles." Even as I say these words, I feel a stab of guilt. Avery is the last child of mine to walk away from me; what's the rush? And yet—walking means freedom, and I want Avery to be free.

Wendy pats my hand. "Remember, development isn't in a straight line. Try not to compare; you wouldn't compare Bennett to Carter. And don't worry. Avery is doing great." Because she says it, and means it, I accept it, and believe it, too.

Ever since the E-LAP with Brittney, Avery likes to put things inside other things. I step into my shoe, only to jam my toe against Wendy's bell-ball. Avery must have moved it while Wendy and I were talking about him.


Bennett climbs out of his crib at night and wanders around the bedroom the boys share, touching the toys, playing in the half dark of the glowing turtle night-light. I can hear him through the wall, the plink of the child-size piano, the whine of the plastic fire truck, the laugh of the stuffed Elmo doll and his singsong "Elmo loves you! Elmo loves you!" When Bennett tires, he climbs in with Avery, who wails and howls at the intrusion until the whole house is awake.

It's time to move Bennett into a real bed—or at least a futon mattress on the floor. Avery will stay in the Pack 'n Play a while longer; but we position it so the mesh window is right next to Bennett's head. That way, they can be close, but Avery can still have his space.

While Tom arranges the furniture, I sort clothes into piles— things that need to be mended, items that are too worn to mend, and clothes that have been outgrown. It's the last category I have trouble with—the little boys are too big for outfits that once were Carter's, so I'm not just letting go of the first set of childhood memories, but the second and third, as well. Some items are too hard to part with: a set of elk-hide booties; a ratty, footed sleeper; a faded patchwork quilt. I set these aside, with no clear idea of what I'll do with them.

I sort through my pregnancy clothes, too—the denim shirt, the black leggings, the cream-colored tunic with the satin ribbon from Phyllis. As I pack up the box, Avery sits at my feet, watching me. It reminds me of when I used to sit on my mother's bed and watch her. An upturned face. Rapt concentration. The pleasure of nearness, a child pulled into a mother's orbit. Soon enough, he'll be too busy for such things.

And it's not just cribs and clothes that are outgrown. When Carter was first beginning to speak, he called birds "cheepcheeps," Popsicles were "posipokes," monsters were "magas." He says all these words correctly, now; it's me who still uses the baby version, particularly when I'm distracted or tired. Bennett says "whee-ha," which is sometimes a noun, meaning a slide or a swing, and other times is a verb—as a warning that he's about to jump or slide or swing—and when I hear it, I run to see what he's doing. Avery says "mmmm" for Mama, "kay" for okay, and "dabu-day," which means I'm happy; it also means Daddy. Avery uses signs, too. "Thank you" is touching your chin with your hand, then moving it away. "Sorry" is a fist tracing a circle over your heart. I use all these phrases and signs without thinking twice. It's a language my children taught me, one they'll someday no longer need, one I'll never forget.

Avery, Bennett, and Carter are watching an "Elmo's World" videotape that we've had since Carter was a baby.

"Elmo's very happy to see you and so is Dorothy," he says from the television screen. "Guess what Elmo is thinking about today?" The littler boys are mesmerized; Carter is watching with six-year-old studiousness.

"That's right, books!" says Elmo.

The video cuts away from Elmo and shows a girl at a library, then a boy reading, then a child sitting on a thick book used as a makeshift booster seat. Two boys wrap a book as a gift. A shelf filled with books, a child drawing in a coloring book.

"How do you read a book?" Elmo asks his pal, Mr. Noodle, who sits on it. A chorus of children's voices answers, "No!" Mr. Noodle puts on his glasses, opens the book, but the children interrupt, "It's upside down!" Poor Mr. Noodle can't get it right, but the children continue to help him. My boys on the couch are laughing and pointing and shouting instructions to the television, too.

The video continues, and there are more shots of children reading and being read to. Dorothy, Elmo's pet goldfish, has a book in her fish tank. A baby in a high chair has a book, too. I notice it's the same message as the *Signing Time!* videos: everyone reads, books are a natural part of everyday life. Elmo's voice is clear and loud, and with the exception that he can't enunciate with his puppet mouth, his manner of speaking reminds me very much of Molly's.

"Elmo's friend Michael went to get a book the other day. He went with his daddy to the library! He taught Elmo all about it!"

The video shows a man with a boy dressed in a dark blue shirt and tan pants. The boy has the same haircut as Carter, same color hair. He wears glasses. The boy and his father look at all sorts of books—about whales, balloons, stories about giants and beanstalks, dinosaurs.

"Michael likes dinosaurs," Elmo says.

*What boy doesn't?* I think.

There's a close-up of Michael, and for a moment I think Michael has Down syndrome. But no, I've seen this video a hundred times. I would have remembered it. I shake it off, laughing at my foolishness—seeing Down syndrome everywhere.

The video shows the library checkout desk, then a home, and we are looking over the boy's shoulder as he sits on his father's lap, reading. I notice the shape of Michael's back, the slope of his shoulders, his neck. Avery's neck. The boy has Down syndrome.

I find the cardboard sleeve of the video and flip to the back, wondering about the people who made it. In small red print, listed under "Writers," is the name Emily Kingsley.

I Google "Emily Perl Kingsley" and learn that she joined the Children's Television Workshop in 1970, which was four years before her son Jason was born with Down syndrome. Her experiences with Jason inspired her to include people with disabilities as a regular part of the *Sesame Street* cast. I learn too that she's spent much of her life working as an advocate for families and people with Down syndrome, and that her son Jason coauthored a book with Mitchell Levitz called, *Count Us In: Growing Up with Down Syndrome.*

A vivid childhood memory comes to me. I'm four years old. The bright morning sun shines through the windows behind the television. I can see dust motes in the shafts of light; to me, they look like sparkles. The brightness makes the television screen seem dark. I have to concentrate to see the images. I'm so filled with happiness I can barely contain myself; it's my favorite show. There's Ernie and Bert, Big Bird and Grover. But the best is the Count. I love to count with the Count.

I've grown up with this show; these images of people of all ages and colors and abilities living and working and playing together. It's possible that I simply didn't need to remember that Michael had Down syndrome, until now. My mind, and heart, is used to the idea of acceptance and inclusion. For this, in part, I have Emily Perl Kingsley to thank.

Once again, she's given me hope. I feel a great sense of relief. It's as if my previous indiscretions—not thinking about the mother or the family of the man at the secondhand store; not knowing what to say to the man gathering shopping carts in the grocery store parking lot—now have a counterpoint. At least there's this: I watched a *Sesame Street* video hundreds of times without focusing on the child with Down syndrome. Before I even knew it mattered, I accepted him without a second thought. If it happened to me, maybe it's happened to other people, too.

Avery and Bennett take a bath together every night. Avery is still a splasher; Bennett no longer gets annoyed, but instead splashes back. It's up to me to intervene, which I do by distracting them with toys, an array of empty yogurt containers, plastic drinking cups, silly straws and bubbles. Avery takes a yogurt container and begins to fill it and empty it. Bennett blows bubbles with the straws.

This is the same tub I leaned against when I woke before sunrise and stumbled into the bathroom, only to find my water had broken. And now here are the babies, grown into toddlers, almost little boys, and my life presses on, all the while moving forward. I absentmindedly hand Avery the clear plastic teddy bear that once held honey; I give Bennett a little green ninja action figure.

The skin around my eyes is lined, where it once was smooth. I have laugh marks around my smile. Hands that look like an old woman's, from so many diaper changes and washings. A pouch of a belly. Feet one size bigger, permanently. These are the reminders; my body tells the story of my life, just as Avery's does, with the crease in the palm of his hand and the stars in his eyes; just as Bennett's does, with the scar at his navel from his surgery.

Watching the boys, I see the way Bennett's body has stretched itself from the chubby, potbellied toddler to the thin, muscular small boy that he is. Avery has a different shape. His body is pearlike: thin legs and arms, a shallow chest, and a big round belly. Bennett has twenty teeth, evenly distributed on top and bottom. Avery has just four, two on top and two on bottom. The top teeth are larger and rounder than Bennett's; the bottom two are thin and pointy. My books have told me to expect Avery's teeth to come in this way, and it doesn't seem to bother him, so it doesn't bother me, either. Instead of seeing what's wrong, I see what's right: with his four teeth, Avery is a terrific eater, and feeds himself with a spoon and fork.

Avery has taken the little green ninja from Bennett. Avery puts the ninja in the plastic teddy bear and smiles, then laughs. The ninja inside the bear! He lifts it up to show me. Laugh laugh laugh. Avery's laugh makes me laugh, too.

"Okay, boys," I say. Then I sign, *All-done,* then, *clean.* Bennett signs, *No,* and when I don't agree, he speaks the word aloud: "No!"

I say, "Yes, it's almost bedtime." I lift each boy from the tub. Bennett runs out of the bathroom and down the hall, streaking though the house. I concentrate on Avery, slathering the Aquaphor all over him, then putting him in a size-three diaper and light blue cotton pajamas decorated with little white puppies. Bennett returns reluctantly, and I grab him and diaper him in a size five. He struggles to put on his own pajamas; I let him try a few times, then intervene. I pick up Avery and lean him against my hip. Taking Bennett by the hand, I lead them out of the bathroom and into the quiet, darkened bedroom.

Bennett settles himself in his bed as I lift Avery into the Pack 'n Play. I kiss each boy good night, then say "I love you" to Bennett.

"Luv," he repeats.

"I love you" to Avery.

He smiles at me, then rolls over.

I turn toward the dresser and twist the knob on a windup toy that plays a lullaby and shines a light show on the walls and ceiling. The dark room brightens and I see giraffes and monkeys and hippos and a lion in a slow-moving parade. I quietly slip away.

Later in the evening, long after the circus parade is over, I hear the familiar, "Elmo loves you! Elmo loves you!" I think maybe Bennett is still awake, so I creep back into the room, only to find that Bennett has climbed into Avery's Pack 'n Play. I leave the boys alone for the moment, and search for the Elmo doll, which has gotten pinned beneath a truck. I free him, and as I do, I notice how threadbare he's become. Our Elmo's fur is no longer furry, but matted from too many washings. His nose is squashed and his right eyeball is scratched. He's my children's version of the Velveteen Rabbit, softened by age and time. Like me, I realize. The better for having been loved.

Avery rolls away from Bennett in his sleep. Avery's little legs are moving, scissoring across the sheet. For an instant, I wonder if he's dreaming, and if in his dreams he can walk.

I remember my dreams as a child—they were so vivid, so real. One in particular began with the wind from *The Wizard of Oz*. I could feel it lift me up, just as it lifted Dorothy's house. I'd rise a little, then float back down to the sidewalk. Again and again, each time lifted higher, until finally I was flying. I never wanted those dreams to end, and I always woke feeling happy.

I think again of Avery and his dreams. I'd imagined he was walking, but as I consider it, I realize I'm not thinking big enough. Maybe, in his dreams, Avery is running. Maybe, in his dreams, he can fly.


Tom and the kids and I drive through the gray spring rain to the local hospital to our doctor's office. The colors of the waiting room—celery and mauve carpeting and upholstery, blond wood—are meant to soothe, but instead they make me edgy. I'm wishing for the red and bright blue and yellow of toys; the comfortable clutter of the boys' room and its litter of fire trucks and wooden train tracks and Duplo blocks. At home, I feel safe.

We register at the front desk, sign release forms, then sit and wait for our names to be called. Time slows like taffy, sticky and fluid. I know it's silly to be so tense. I've lived with these boys every moment of their waking lives since they came home from the NICU, and I've come to know them. I know they're healthy. I know they're strong. I know this, and yet I doubt it. I need to hear it from someone else. I'm waiting for our doctor to give me permission to stop being afraid.

The boys' second birthday is a reckoning of sorts—the end of the adjusted ages, the end of prematurity. I worry that for Avery there will be something more, something new. It's a worry that's always there, even on the brightest day, like a shadow at high noon, waiting for the slanting light to reveal itself. We missed so many troubles—heart issues, problems with vision, thyroid imbalance, hearing impairment. No RSV, no pneumonia. Surely, it's time for more rough water.

Part of me realizes I'm being irrational; I held on to fear so tightly for so long, I can't let go of it. And I wonder, too, if it's guilt. I didn't appreciate Avery quickly enough, which means I'll lose him—it's right that I should. A mother who's been given a pearl and doesn't appreciate it doesn't deserve it.

I have time to think of all of this while waiting for our names to be called, and more time still. I chase Bennett around the chair in a hundred circles; I play peek-a-boo with Avery for a thousand years, when finally I hear, "Avery and Bennett?"

A nurse leads us to an exam room for more waiting. Carter shifts in the one chair and says, "I'm bored, Mom." *Where did he learn such an expression?* I hand him a *Ranger Rick*. Tom and the babies and I sit on the floor.

"Cool, Mom, look at this," Carter says, then shows me a photo of a lime green fish with a dozen eggs in its mouth. "It's how the mother fish protects them." I envy the mother fish. I wish I could gather up my children and hold them inside me and protect them forever.

"They should play music in the waiting rooms," Tom says. "Something happy. Like polka. It's all so serious." He knows how worried I am, and he's trying to be reassuring.

When our doctor arrives, he seems a little older than the last time we saw him. He has a few more gray hairs at his temple, and he's thinner. The key is gone from around his neck. He asks how we've been, and he tells Tom that he enjoyed reading his book. Tom nods and mumbles, "Thanks."

Pleasantries aside, the doctor begins his examinations, Bennett first. He pauses at Bennett's belly button, the site of the surgery.

"This has healed nicely," the doc says.

He looks into Bennett's eyes, his ears. Bennett tolerates all the pushing and prodding with a mild curiosity. He's come so far—a baby who started life with the temperament of a grouchy old man; now, most of the time, he's happy.

Avery is next. The doctor looks into his eyes, his ears. He feels his tummy, his sides, his scrotum. The doc touches a stethoscope to the palm of his hand to warm it, then listens to Avery's heart. He pulls Avery's legs together and looks at his knees; then he runs the palm of his hand over the soles of Avery's little feet.

He takes more care with Avery than he did with Bennett, and he handles him more gently, but this time, it doesn't bother me. I look at Avery's naked body—so much bigger than it used to be, yet still so small. Avery's soft skin. His hair, the color of ripe wheat. His blue eyes, like his brothers', like mine.

I remember the feel of his head tucked beneath my chin when he was a baby. His tiny starfish hand, opening and closing. Holding him close, dancing to Nina Simone as raindrops slid down the windowpane. Soft, papery skin. Sweet, wet kisses. His little face at the foot of my bed, watching me get dressed, playing with my socks.

The doctor nods for me to put Avery back in his diaper and clothes. My hands are unsteady and I fumble with the Velcro tabs on the diaper as if I were a new mom all over again. The doctor tells us to make sure Avery has a low-fat, high-fiber diet. I slip Avery's head into his shirt; he pokes his hands through the arms on his own. The doctor reminds us to get the blood work done for Avery's periodic thyroid check. I pull up Avery's pants. The doctor suggests that we select a dentist. I slip on Avery's socks, tie his shoes. The doctor tells us to come back when Avery's three.

I continue listening. Avery is dressed. I wait quietly for the bad news.

Finally the doctor says, "Okay, then," and begins gathering up the file folders.

"That's it?" I ask.

"Yes. Unless you have any questions?"

"Everything's okay?" I repeat.

"Yes," he says. "Everything is great."


I belong to a group called Wild Horse Writers, consisting of a dozen people who meet once a month in the conference room of the public library to discuss our works in progress, mostly poetry and prose. We're an eclectic bunch, with a wide range of interests, including Christianity, vampires, holistic health, Chinese dragons, Montana history, photography, mindful meditation, maple trees, and Down syndrome. We are pro-life and pro-choice; we are Republican and Democrat; we are married, divorced, remarried, never married, and single. We are parents and we are childless; we are eleven women and one man. What keeps us together is a shared sense of creativity, and the desire to support one another in telling our stories.

When it's my turn to read, I cry my way through a short little paragraph I'd written about Avery's birth. The power of my feelings, even two years later, stuns me. It's as if no time has passed, and I'm back at the lake, floating. Arms extended, feet spread, my own Vitruvian man balanced on the water by surface tension and the rise and fall of my own breath. The only sound is my heartbeat, steady like a drum.

When the meeting concludes, a woman named Mary asks if I'll go with her to her car, so she can give me something. I don't know much about Mary, except that her writing is lyric and flowing and beautiful, and that she is a healer. She helps people understand the language of their bodies.

Mary and I say our good-byes to the other group members, and I follow her across the street to her car. From the backseat she pulls out a basket filled with tiny glass bottles. She asks my permission to proceed, and I say yes. She closes her eyes and begins her communication, but it's not a language of speech, or a language of signs; it's a language of body movements and shifts within her.

She opens her eyes, reaches into the basket, and pulls out a bottle. She asks if she can touch me, and again, I say yes. She dabs some of the liquid from the bottle on her index finger, then taps each of my earlobes. I'm enveloped in fragrance—the white lilacs blooming in the moonlight. The heady peonies. Sun-dried cotton pillowcases. My grandmother's kitchen in the mornings.

"What is it?" I ask.

"Forgiveness," she says.

It is the one, perfect word. I crack. Tears flow out of me like a river flowing to the ocean. I have so much guilt. I was too old to have a baby. Or it's deeper within me, a rotten core of bad genes that Avery has to pay for. My selfishness, my doubt. It all comes pouring out.

"I was so afraid," I say. "I was so scared. He could be held by anyone; and so I let him. He was everybody's baby but my own."

Mary is quiet, listening to me with her whole body, listening the way the grass hears the rain. As I tell her my story, I can feel the sadness lift from my body, replaced by a newborn tenderness. It is forgiveness, for Avery, and for me.

"Would you like to walk over to the water?" she asks.

I nod yes. We walk side by side down the slope toward the water's edge. Here, the air is wet and cool and sweet. It's as if I am breathing for the first time, and it feels good. I feel good.

We sit together, watching the lights of the cars cross the bridge in the distance. Out of the corner of my eye I think I see a bright burst of color. A moment later there is another *pop* and a *kaboom*, followed by the unmistakable sizzle of fireworks and more *kabooms!* and *pops!* and shooting stars, bursting open with great explosions. I look at Mary, who merely shrugs and smiles, as if she were used to light shows following her around. I feel free, and giddy. I laugh.

When the fireworks end, the silence is round and full and perfect like the moon as it rises over the mountains to the east. I can't think of any reason for there to be fireworks on an ordinary Thursday evening, a night like any other, except on this night, I was forgiven.

# 14

## Parting Gifts

The day is so full of summer that the sun shining on the water makes the lake appear to be full of diamonds. Seagulls dive and swoop overhead. Bennett calls them eagles. The ice cream stand next to the playground is doing a brisk business. Avery signs, *Ice cream?*

*Wait,* I sign back.

Bennett rushes ahead to the slide. The apparatus is made of red metal stairs, a hinged walkway, and a blue plastic slide. We've been meeting Wendy here for physical therapy. The change gives Avery a chance to work on playground skills, though to him and Bennett, it just seems like fun.

Avery sinks down to his bottom and scoots away from me. I rush after him, but Wendy gets there first. She picks up Avery and holds him until he drops his legs and begins trying to walk. He takes a few reluctant, supported steps.

"Good work, Avery!" she says cheerfully.

We have our routine: She puts Avery's hands on the railing, and prompts him to take the first step, then the second. I duck beneath the slide and come out on the other side, to block an opening meant for bigger kids. Wendy guides Avery past it and I move to the bottom of the slide, to catch Avery as he tumbles out. Then I support him as he walks over to the stairs, and we repeat the process.

I bend beneath the slide, and as I straighten I see a vehicle I recognize pulling into the parking lot, a black Suburban. The back doors spread and children climb out. An older boy runs toward us and shouts, "Hi, Jennifer." He's grown taller, and his hair is in his eyes. He has the same goofy smile; the same, uneven way of getting your attention. All the other kids call me "Carter's Mom," but he's always called me "Jennifer." Cathy's son.

He joins me, curious. He wants to know which boy is which, and I tell him. He wants to know why we're here, and I say we're here to play. He wants to know where Carter is, and I tell him he's at home, with his dad. He asks why Avery can't walk.

"He will walk," I say, "but he needs to practice. We're helping him, and you can help him, too." Other kids have crowded around, listening.

"Why can't he talk?" another asks.

"He can talk," I say, "a little bit. But sometimes, he also talks with his hands. It's called sign language."

I show the children the sign for *walk*, which is two fingers walking on the palm of the hand. I also show them the sign for *ice cream*, which looks as if you're holding and licking an imaginary ice cream cone. I've missed the switch to my post at the bottom of the slide, but Wendy covers for me. All the children seem to be having fun, Avery included.

Cathy waves from a distance. She's bypassed the play equipment, walking in an arc to avoid it, and is standing near the water. She calls for her son. He tells me, "I have to go. Good-bye, Jennifer!" and runs to his mother. A few children follow him. They begin throwing rocks in the lake.

*All kids like to throw rocks in the lake*, I think. But I know better. She told her son and his friends to stay away from us.

*Maybe she wanted to give us room to work*, I think. *Maybe she wanted to help.*

We don't need that kind of help. We need to be seen, we need to be heard, we need to be included. Her son could see this; why couldn't she?

*Let it go*, I tell myself. It's a relief to turn back to Avery and resume my place in our routine, catching him at the bottom of the slide, his laughing face turned up toward me, his arms stretched wide.

Two other mothers have drifted over from the ice cream shack. Their children join us, and I explain again what we are doing, and again, I teach a few signs. It's a summer day. The lake is sparkling. Seagulls soar and dip on the breeze. Some of the children stayed back with us. The sun keeps shining, and the seagulls see us from above, and from a seagull's point of view, we are all of a kind, just children and mommies, playing together.

Avery wakes before his brothers. He gets himself out of bed, quietly opens the door, and scoots down the hall to find me. He hugs me—wrapping his thin, strong arms around me, burying his face in my hair—and then the day can begin.

Each morning I crack brown eggs into a white ceramic bowl, two for two little boys, sometimes three, one for me. Carter used to eat eggs for breakfast; now he prefers peanut butter on whole wheat toast. I pour the eggs into a hot cast-iron pan that once belonged to my great-grandmother and stir the yolks, watching the yellow spread like sunshine.

I take out an empty cooking pot and hand Avery a few pieces of uncooked macaroni. He puts the macaroni in the pot carefully, one at a time, *pink plink plink*. I give him a blue plastic spoon and the lid to the pot, too. He works at my feet, cooking, while I finish making breakfast. By the time the eggs are ready, and the toast, Carter and Bennett are awake, too.

Carter sits at the table in front of the big window that looks out across the lake. Bennett likes to sit next to him, and copies whatever Carter does. Avery goes in the high chair, because he tolerates it, and I feel safer with him there. Soon enough, though, he's going to want to sit in a big chair. The boys eat and I drink coffee and look out at a lone kayak making its way to one of the islands. The morning is cool yet, but I can feel the heat of the day rising with the sun.

The stack of paperwork on top of the microwave has thinned. Avery's therapy bills are paid through the new insurance; once a month, we get a statement listing all the services he's received, and I file that away in a dark blue binder. On the fridge, there's a regular calendar, with playdates written in, and birthdays, and holidays. No more urgent messages, or emergency phone numbers, or feeding charts. I still have a little pad of paper for keeping notes, but now it's full of things like grocery lists or story ideas.

Avery must have noticed me scribbling in my little notebook, because he loves to draw. I find his scribbles in board books, and in places where he thinks I might not notice: on the floor beneath a corner of the rug, on the white wall behind the curtain, on the side of the wooden rocking horse that's usually against the wall. I don't know where he gets the pens, the pencils, the markers, the crayons—I try to keep them out of reach—but Avery has a way of finding them.

He's interested in the computer, too, more so than Bennett. Avery sits at my feet and signs, *more!* or *please!,* and if I don't respond, he says, "Psst," or "Mmaaa!" until I pick him up and sit him in my lap. He likes to look at pictures of other children. Online communities like Downsyn.com, and T21 Online, and Uno Mas! and BabyCenter.com have message boards where posters can add signature pictures, or build photo galleries. Here, children are everywhere. Little boys Avery might befriend; little girls he might someday marry. A community full of people like us—mothers, fathers, sisters, brothers—with faces that look like family.

I'm washing the last bit of eggs from the cast-iron pan when the kids' videotape ends and pops out of the machine. The television is on; it's *Good Morning America*. Onscreen, a young man is talking about his recent research concerning the prenatal diagnosis of Down syndrome. He's handsome, and speaks kindly about babies with Down syndrome and mothers of babies with Down syndrome. Not surprisingly, I decide I like him right away.

His name is Brian Skotko and he's a student at the Harvard Medical School and the Kennedy School. As part of his coursework, Skotko mailed an eleven-page survey to nearly three thousand members of five Down syndrome parent organizations in California, Colorado, Massachusetts, North Carolina, and Rhode Island, requesting information about each mother's experience with prenatal diagnosis.

From the responses, Skotko learned that the women felt their doctors didn't tell them about the positive potential of people with Down syndrome; they didn't receive enough up-to-date information about the condition; and they weren't often given connections to other parents. The mothers in the survey felt this lack of support happens at a critical time, when many women are trying to decide if they will continue their pregnancies. Skotko's survey is the largest and most comprehensive study on prenatal diagnosis of Down syndrome to date.

The television interview ends, but I want to know more. I Google "Brian Skotko" and learn that based on the comments from his survey, Skotko created seven recommendations for anyone delivering a diagnosis of Down syndrome. I read through the points.

"Results from the prenatal screening should be clearly explained as a risk assessment, not as a 'positive' or 'negative' result." *Yes*, I think, this is fair. "Results from the amniocentesis or CVS should, whenever possible, be delivered in person with both parents present." Again, *Yes*. This suggestion is clear. "Sensitive language should be used when delivering a diagnosis of Down syndrome." Again, obvious. "If obstetricians rely on genetic counselors or other specialists to explain Down syndrome, sensitive, accurate, and consistent messages must be conveyed." And I think, *Yes, yes, of course. What's so earth-shaking about these requests?*

Skotko's "Seven Talking Points" are a decent, gentle way of communicating a medical fact, without judgment or implication. I find myself beginning to cry. In my mind, this conversation is not about a theoretical baby; it's about Avery. These are such basic rights, a way of speaking about my son with simple human dignity. It saddens me that Skotko's points aren't already commonplace.

The recommendations continue: "Physicians should discuss all reasons for prenatal diagnosis, including reassurance, advance awareness before delivery of the diagnosis of Down syndrome, adoption, as well as pregnancy termination," and "Up-to-date information on Down syndrome should be available," and finally, "Contact with local Down syndrome support groups should be offered, if desired."

I think back on my own experience. What if we'd known about Avery, and had been told the very worst, been given the grimmest outlook, and then been offered the solution of abortion? I know how I would have felt. I would have felt scared. I would have felt as if I'd done something wrong. I would have felt alone. We can't know the power of forgiveness until we have experienced it ourselves. We can't know the power of love, either. I don't want to live in a world without both—forgiveness and love.

I'm wearing a red-and-white-striped shirt and blue jeans—Tom says I look like the American flag. I make a space for the paper napkins on a glass table that's filled with food—bratwurst and chicken-apple sausages, potato chips, watermelon. There are glass bottles of cherry vanilla soda and root beer, from the brewery in town. Judith, a woman from my writing group, has brought coffee chocolate brownies, and Judith's daughter Emily made a tomato and mozzarella salad. Emily and her husband, Vince, also brought a Slip 'n Slide for the boys, their first one. The sun is warm, the lake is calm and smooth, the mountains are green. The air smells of pine and roses, from the clusters of deep red blooms on the bush behind the house.

For the party, we set up tables in the back, behind the house, and we moved the grill there, too. Don is cooking the brats and the chicken sausages. Joyce is in the kitchen. Tom's older brother, Bob, and his wife, Elizabeth, are visiting from Boulder, Colorado. They have two children, Daniel, who is a year and a half older than Carter, and Gracie, who's Carter's age. They're in town for the Fourth of July, and then they plan to spend a few days in Glacier National Park.

Tom blocked off the driveway with sawhorses to make room for chairs and picnic umbrellas. People park at the bottom of the hill and drift up to the house. I see Sarah, wearing a tie-dyed summer dress, with Ric and their two boys. Michelle and Eric, their little boy Braden, and their new baby, Kenna. Friends from the fire department, neighbors. Tom's friend Bob brought his accordion.

A line of kids races past me—Daniel is in the lead, then Carter and Gracie. Bennett slows at the table, snatches a potato chip, then runs to catch up with the others. I'm reminded of my own childhood, and my parents' parties, and how my sister and I used to sit beneath the table, hidden by the tablecloth, and listen to the adults' conversations. We'd take turns darting out to retrieve plates of snacks: tiny pizzas, rye cocktail rounds topped with cheddar cheese spread, mini pigs in a blanket.

My sister-in-law's mother is from Spain, and Elizabeth is bilingual. She speaks Spanish to Avery and tells me, "I know he understands!" and calls him *my dear, my love, my sweet.* Judith holds Avery, then Emily. Sarah, then Michelle. Avery doesn't mind; in fact, he's a little bit of a flirt. He gives each new face his biggest, brightest smile. He makes his sounds, he blows raspberries; then he breaks out his best skill—he hums "Itsy Bitsy Spider" and shows off the hand movements he's learned. When he's finished, he claps for himself.

After supper, Tom's friend Bob plays an improvised song on his accordion: "Gracie and the Pink Shoes." All the children want personalized songs; they form a small half-moon at Bob's feet. Avery sits right in the middle.

When the show is over, I find myself speaking with a woman I haven't met before, the date of a friend of Tom's. She tells me about her life in Seattle, and how she's always wanted to visit Montana. She's never been married; she has no children. Her career is her life, but she tells me she's thinking of making a change. I nod sympathetically, then begin telling her about my life, specifically about Avery, and as I'm speaking, I realize I've crossed over into a new place. I have a new feeling about it all. I think for a moment, and it surprises me.

"It's okay," I say, and change the subject.

For once, I don't feel the need to explain myself. I have all the words; and now that I do, I don't need to use them. It's a party, after all. The night is filled with the sound of voices and laughter. A fuss breaks out among the children—someone was pushing someone else down the hill on the wagon, too fast. A few of the dads split up the kids and settle the argument, then redirect everyone's attention to the glow sticks and sparklers and the stars that are just beginning to come out.

For a brief moment, I wonder who I might have been, if Carter was my only child. I probably would be worrying about the food, or my clothes. I'd be thinking small thoughts, little unimportant ones, and I'd miss the big picture. I feel it anew, in every cell of my body: the voices, the laughter. I see it: the beauty of the faces of the children holding sparklers. Fathers and mothers bent over them from behind, supporting them, guiding them. Everyone lustrous and shining.

I think again of the nine-out-of-ten statistic, only this time, I also think about the women who might choose a child like Avery. I see them all around me: these are the women I pin my hopes on. These are the mothers of our future, if the future is to include children like Avery.

The *pskt pskt pskt* of the automatic sprinkler sends water arcing out over the garden in rainbows. Avery, Bennettt, Carter, Tom, and I are all together on the green slope of grass in front of the gate. Avery is putting rocks into the yellow plastic watering can, one at a time. Bennett plays with a metal Tonka truck full of gravel. Carter is helping Tom unroll the yellow plastic Slip 'n Slide.

What I expect will happen is that Mr. Whee-ha (Bennett) will love the Slip 'n Slide. Carter, too. But Avery won't go for it; he'll want to keep close to me. Tom blows air into the dark blue plastic bumpers that line the slide and form a shallow splash pool at the end. I remind the boys of the rules, "Remember, one at a time. Take turns."

Tom pushes the plastic pegs through the four tags on the slide down into the grass. He attaches the green garden hose and the plastic expands like a party balloon filling with air. At first, there's only a fine mist, but it quickly grows and we all get sprayed. The water is cool and drops catch on my eyelashes. Laughter, shouts of glee. Tom runs to the faucet and adjusts it.

Carter knows what to do. He takes a running leap onto the slide, and turns himself into a long, lean streak slipping through the water. He screams and squeals with delight.

Next, it's Bennett's turn. I urge him on with a "Go, Benny! Go!" But instead of running up the hill to the slide, Mr. Whee-ha runs to me and buries his face in my chest. Tom looks over to see if I need help. I shake my head, *We're okay*.

Avery begins scooting up to the top of the slide. I see it happening as if in slow motion—me, holding Bennett in my arms. Tom trying to catch Avery. Carter, running across the lawn to get to Avery, too. But before we can reach him, Avery launches himself into the spray.

He flops down on his belly and pedals with his arms, swooshing through the water, licking at the air. He's smiling, a wide, happy grin that spreads across his whole face, laughing all the way down the slide. In the little pool of water at the bottom, he lingers, splashing. We're all there, now. Around him. Avery claps for himself, hooray!

Carter laughs, Tom and me, too, from relief that Avery's okay, and from amazement, at his ability and his fearlessness. Even Bennett seems heartened. While we're laughing, Avery scoots up to the top of the slide, to take another turn. Avery, our little seal pup, sliding and smiling, happy and free.


Later in the evening, when the Slip 'n Slide has been rolled up and packed away, when the sprinklers have been turned off and the hoses looped back into coils, the only sounds are the lapping of the water on the lake and an occassional motorboat heading to shore. The kids have eaten a supper of macaroni and cheese and green beans and chocolate milk. Carter is allowed to stay up for an extra half hour to play a computer game.

The little boys are already in bed; they've had their bedtime stories and brushed their teeth and had one last drink of water. I turn toward the dresser and twist the knob on the toy that plays the lullaby and shines the light show on the walls and ceiling. The dark room brightens with giraffes and monkeys and hippos. I make sure Avery has his stuffed puppy, Bennett his little monkey. I kiss each good night, then say, "I love you" to Bennett.

"Luv you," he repeats.

"I love you" to Avery.

I turn toward the door, when I hear a soft voice that I don't recognize.

"Ahluvyou."

I swing around, and Avery is smiling at me.

I go to him. I kiss him on the forehead. "Good boy, Avery," I say, with tears in my eyes. "Mommy loves you so much."

I find Tom and can barely speak. I manage to get my point across and he follows me back into the bedroom, hoping to hear for himself.

"Love you, Avery," Tom says.

It's difficult for Avery to manage again—this time he says it too loud and the words come out in a rush, "Ahluvyou!"

The musical lullaby light is playing, the stars of the slow-moving parade circle around us. I can see tears in Tom's eyes. It's one moment in time, silver and perfect, shining and whole. It's a gift, from Avery to us, of what he has to give: his love.


My friend Claudia prays each morning. She talks to God as if he were a close friend, a personal confidant. I've never been able to do that, though I wish I could. When I pray, words are hard to come by.

I call Claudia and ask her to help me.

I tell her the parts of my story that I've never told anyone— the *meaningful hug* from Sandy B. and the feeling of being surrounded by love, of being held in the cup of the palm of a hand. I explain about the first *woo-woo card*, and how I felt love for Tom and the boys so purely that it took away all of my anger. And the second *woo-woo card*, when I was afraid, and it told me to have courage. The third one—the Lord's prayer. Only now, when I look at them, they're just cards. They don't work anymore. I ask her why it had to go away.

"I don't think it did go away," she says gently. "I think it's been there all along, and maybe you just stopped paying attention."

As soon as she says it, I know she's right.

When I was a girl, I received an award for perfect attendance at Summer Vacation Bible School. The prize was a button with a cartoon frog on it and the words "Who you are is your gift from God. What you make of yourself is your gift to God." I lived with that button hanging from the light cord in my closet for most of my young life. Each time I pulled on the light, I touched it. Each time I turned off the light, I touched it again. And yet despite my familiarity with it, I don't think I understood what it meant until now: I'm part of the circle, too.

If it's true that God hears our prayers, he answers them with things like the slip of paper from the nurse with Robby's mom's phone number on it, or Brittney's coffee can. A windmill alongside the highway, or a sparkly three-star barrette unearthed in the garden dirt, or fireworks in the middle of June.

He answers prayers in kindness that circulates from one person to another. Tom, Carter, Avery, and Bennett are a part of the circle. And Tom's folks, and mine. Sarah and Phyllis and Claudia. And my teachers, Wendy and Brittney and Molly and Mary, who helped me learn how to find my own way, not by doing it for me, but by allowing me to do it for myself.

We live in a house at the end of a twisty gravel road, on a hilltop overlooking a lake. There are words on the walls, hidden beneath the paint. Things like "sunshine" and "happiness," "music" and "books" and "love."

At our house, people take off their shoes and leave them in a line by the door. When no one's watching, Avery tucks his favorite things into the empty shoes, like parting gifts—the Matchbox fire truck, the little green ninja, his blue spoon. Despite the startled guests and the stubbed toes, it's hard for me to be mad at him. He's the child that I wanted, that I did not know I wanted.

He is my son.

# Chapter Notes

### 1    At First, It Hurts to Breathe

Cohen, William I., Lynn Nadel, and Myra E. Madnick, eds. *Down Syndrome: Visions for the 21st Century.* New York: Wiley-Liss, Inc., 2002.

### 2    Slipping

Agnew, Connie, Allen H. Klein, et al. *Twins!: Expert Advice from Two Practicing Physicians on Pregnancy, Birth, and the First Year of Life with Twins.* New York: HarperCollins Publishers, 1997.

Luke, Barbara, and Tamara Eberlein. *When You're Expecting Twins, Triplets, or Quads: A Complete Resource.* New York: HarperCollins Publishers, 1999.

### 3    Please, Come Back to Me

Cohen, Nadel, and Madnick, eds. *Down Syndrome.*

Klein, Stanley, Ph.D., and Kim Schive, eds. *You Will Dream New Dreams: Inspiring Personal Stories by Parents of Children with Disabilities.* New York: Kensington Books, 2001.

NDSS. "Down Syndrome: Myths and Truths." New York: National Down Syndrome Society, 1999.

Stray-Gundersen, Karen, ed. *Babies with Down Syndrome: A New Parents' Guide*, 2nd ed. Bethesda, MD: Woodbine House, 1995.

## 4    Home Is Not Where You Thought It Was

Astoria, Dorothy. *The Name Book*. Minneapolis: Bethany House Publishers, 1997.

Cunningham, Cliff. *Understanding Down Syndrome: An Introduction for Parents*. Cambridge, MA: Brookline Books, 1996.

MPRRC. "A Primer on People First Language." Logan, UT: Mountain Plains Regional Resource Center, 1999.

Pueschel, Siegfried M. *A Parent's Guide to Down Syndrome: Toward a Brighter Future*. Baltimore: Paul H. Brookes Publishing Co., 1990.

Stray-Gundersen, ed. *Babies with Down Syndrome*.

Wormser, Richard. *Hoboes: Wandering in America, 1870–1940*. New York: Walker & Company, 1994.

## 5    Caffeine

La Leche League International. *The Womanly Art of Breastfeeding*, 6th rev. ed. Schaumburg, IL: La Leche League International, 1997.

Meyer, D. J., ed. *Uncommon Fathers: Reflections on Raising a Child with a Disability*. Rockville, MD: Woodbine House, 1995.

Stray-Gundersen, ed. *Babies with Down Syndrome*.

Van Dyke, D. C., Philip Mattheis, Susan Schoon Eberly, and Janet Williams, eds. *Medical and Surgical Care for Children with Down Syndrome: A Guide for Parents*. Bethesda, MD: Woodbine House, 1995.

## 6    Cathy Can't Handle Us

Brazelton, T. Berry. *Touchpoints: Your Child's Emotional and Behavioral Development.* Reading, MA: Addison-Wesley Publishing Co., 1992.

Cunningham. *Understanding Down Syndrome.*

Pueschel. *A Parent's Guide to Down Syndrome.*

SSA. "SSA-3820-BK Disability Report—Child"; "SSA-3375-BK Function Report"; "Authorization to Disclose Information to the Social Security Administration." Baltimore, MD: Social Security Administration, 2003.

Stray-Gundersen, ed. *Babies with Down Syndrome.*

## 7    They All Do That

Leshin, Len. "Down Syndrome: Health Issues, News and Information for Parents and Professionals," 1997–present; www.ds-health.com/.

NDSS. "A Promising Future Together: A Guide for New and Expectant Parents." New York: National Down Syndrome Society, 2003.

Stray-Gundersen, ed. *Babies with Down Syndrome.*

Van Dyke, Mattheis, et al., eds. *Medical and Surgical Care for Children with Down Syndrome.*

## 8    I Think I Remember

Beck, Martha. *Expecting Adam: A True Story of Birth, Rebirth and Everyday Magic.* New York: Crown Publishing Group, 1998.

Bérubé, Michael. *Life As We Know It: A Father, a Family, and an Exceptional Child.* New York: Knopf, 1996.

Britt, David W., Samantha T. Risinger, et al. "Determinants of Parental Decisions After the Prenatal Diagnosis of Down

Syndrome: Bringing in Context." *American Journal of Medical Genetics*, 1999.

Gill, Barbara. *Changed by a Child: Companion Notes for Parents of a Child with a Disability*. Garden City, NY: Doubleday, 1997.

*Glover, N. M., and S. J. Glover.* "Ethical and Legal Issues Regarding Selective Abortion of Fetuses with Down Syndrome." *Mental Retardation*, 1996.

Mansfield, Caroline, Sue Hopfer, and Theresa M. Marteau. "Termination Rates After Prenatal Diagnosis of Down Syndrome, Spina Bifida, Anencephaly, and Turner and Klinefelter Syndromes: A Systematic Literature Review." *Prenatal Diagnosis* 19 (1999), pp. 808–12.

Noble, Vicki. *Down Is Up for Aaron Eagle: A Mother's Spiritual Journey with Down Syndrome*. New York: HarperCollins, 1993.

Parens, Erik, and Adrienne Asch. "Disability Rights Critique of Prenatal Genetic Testing: Reflections and Recommendations." *Mental Retardation and Developmental Disabilities Research Reviews*, 2003.

Rothman, Barbara Katz. *The Book of Life: A Personal and Ethical Guide to Race, Normality, and the Implications of the Human Genome Project*. Boston: Beacon Press, 2000.

Stray-Gundersen, ed. *Babies with Down Syndrome*.

Thomas, Marlo. *Free to Be . . . You and Me*. Audio CD, original recording remastered, Arista, 2006.

Trainer, Marilyn. *Differences in Common: Straight Talk on Mental Retardation, Down Syndrome, and Life*. Bethesda, MD: Woodbine House, 1991.

Will, George. "Eugenics by Abortion: Is Perfection an Entitlement?" *Washington Post*, April 14, 2005.

Vredevelt, Pam. *Angel Behind the Rocking Chair.* New York: Waterbrook Press, 1998.


## 9    Some Days Are Better Than Others

Carver, Raymond. *A New Path to the Waterfall: Poems.* New York: Grove/Atlantic, 1989.

Cunningham. *Understanding Down Syndrome.*

Leshin. "Down Syndrome."

MacLeod, Kent. *Down Syndrome and Vitamin Therapy.* Baltimore: Kemanso Publishing Ltd., 2003.

Medlen, Joan Guthrie. *The Down Syndrome Nutrition Handbook: A Guide to Promoting Healthy Lifestyles.* Lake Oswego, OR: Phronesis Publishing, 2006.

NuTriVene-D Targeted Nutritional Intervention, A Brand of International Nutrition, Inc.; www.nutrivene.com/.

Pueschel. *A Parent's Guide to Down Syndrome.*

Stray-Gundersen, ed. *Babies with Down Syndrome.*

Sumar, Sonia. *Yoga for the Special Child: A Therapeutic Approach for Infants and Children with Down Syndrome, Cerebral Palsy, and Learning Disabilities.* Buckingham, VA: Special Yoga Publications, 1998.

Wenig, Marsha. *YogaKids: An Easy, Fun-filled Adventure.* DVD; Living Arts, Inc., 2000.


## 10    Alphabet Soup

Bricker, Diane, et al. *Ages & Stages Questionnaires (ASQ).* Baltimore: Paul H. Brookes Publishing Co., 1995.

Child Development Center (CDC); www.childdevcenter.org/.

Coleman, Jeanine G. *The Early Intervention Dictionary: A Multidisciplinary Guide to Terminology.* Bethesda, MD: Woodbine House, 1993.

Cunningham. *Understanding Down Syndrome.*

Glover, M. E., J. L. Preminger, and A. R. Sanford. *Early LAP: The Early Learning Accomplishment Profile for Young Children, Birth to 36 Months.* Chapel Hill, NC: Chapel Hill Training-Outreach Project, 1988.

Marino, B., and Siegfried M. Pueschel, eds. *Heart Disease in Persons with Down Syndrome.* Baltimore: Paul H. Brookes, 1996.

National Down Syndrome Society (NDSS); www.ndss.org/.

Pueschel. *A Parent's Guide to Down Syndrome.*

Schermerhorn, Will. *Down Syndrome: The First 18 Months.* DVD; Vienna, VA: Blueberry Shoes Productions, 1993.

Stray-Gundersen, ed. *Babies with Down Syndrome.*

## 11   Taxi Rides

Bruni, Maryanne. *Fine Motor Skills for Children with Down Syndrome: A Guide for Parents and Professionals.* Bethesda, MD: Woodbine House, 1998.

Cohen, Nadel, and Madnick, eds. *Down Syndrome.*

da Vinci, Leonardo. *The Vitruvian Man.* Pen and ink drawing; available at http://leonardodavinci.stanford.edu/submissions/clabaugh/history/leonardo.html; accessed April 5, 2007.

Jobling, Anne, and Naznin Virji-Babul. *Down Syndrome: Play, Move, and Grow.* Vancouver, BC: Down Syndrome Research Foundation, 2004.

Pueschel. *A Parent's Guide to Down Syndrome.*

Schermerhorn. *Down Syndrome.*

Simone, Nina. *Little Girl Blue.* LP; "My Baby Just Cares for Me," recording studio session, 1957, New York. Gus Kahn, Walter Donaldson, extended version.

Winders, Patricia C. *Gross Motor Skills in Children with Down Syndrome: A Guide for Parents and Professionals.* Bethesda, MD: Woodbine House, 1997.

12    More, More

Cohen, Nadel, and Madnick, eds. *Down Syndrome.*

Coleman, Rachel. *Signing Time! Volume 1: My First Signs.* VHS & DVD; Salt Lake City: Two Little Hands Productions, 2002.

Kaiser, A., and D. Gray, eds. *Enhancing Children's Communication: Research Foundations for Intervention.* Baltimore: Paul H. Brookes Publishing Co., 1993.

Kumin, Libby. *Early Communication Skills for Children with Down Syndrome: A Guide for Parents and Professionals.* Bethesda, MD: Woodbine House, 2003.

Pueschel. *A Parent's Guide to Down Syndrome.*

Riski, Maureen, and Nikolas Klakow. *Oliver Gets Hearing Aids.* Warrenville, IL: Harrison Communications, 2001.

Schermerhorn. *Down Syndrome.*

Schwartz, Susan, and Joan E. Heller Miller. *The New Language of Toys: Teaching Communication Skills to Children with Special Needs, A Guide for Parents and Teachers.* Bethesda, MD: Woodbine House, 1996.

Stray-Gundersen, ed. *Babies with Down Syndrome.*

Van Dyke, Mattheis, et al., eds. *Medical and Surgical Care for Children with Down Syndrome.*

13    Everybody's Baby but My Own

Children's Television Workshop. *Sesame Street, Elmo's World: Dancing, Music and Books.* VHS; directed by Emily Squires and Ted May, manufactured by Sony Wonder, a division of Sony Music, New York, 2000.

Cohen, Nadel, and Madnick, eds. *Down Syndrome.*

Coleman, Rachel. *Signing Time! Volume 2: Playtime Signs.* VHS & DVD; Salt Lake City: Two Little Hands Productions, 2002.

———. *Signing Time! Volume3: Everyday Signs.* VHS & DVD; Salt Lake City: Two Little Hands Productions, 2002.

Kingsley, Emily Perl; www.imdb.com/name/nm0455513/; accessed April 5, 2007.

Kingsley, Jason, and Mitchell Levitz. *Count Us In: Growing Up with Down Syndrome.* New York: Harcourt, 2007.

National Down Syndrome Society (NDSS); www.ndss.org/.

Van Dyke, Mattheis, et al., eds. *Medical and Surgical Care for Children with Down Syndrome.*

Winders. *Gross Motor Skills.*

## 14    Parting Gifts

Baby Center Bulletin Boards, Down Syndrome; http://boards .babycenter.com/n/pfx/forum.aspx?webtag=bcus11985/.

DownSyn Forum; www.downsyn.com/.

Falvey, M. *Believe in My Child with Special Needs!: Helping Children Achieve Their Potential in School.* Baltimore: Brookes Publishing, 2005.

Oelwein, P. *Teaching Reading to Children with Down Syndrome: A Guide for Parents and Teachers.* Bethesda, MD: Woodbine House, 1995.

Pitzer, Marjorie W. *I Can, Can You?* Bethesda, MD: Woodbine House, 2004.

Rickert, Janet Elizabeth. *Russ and the Firehouse.* Bethesda, MD: Woodbine House, 1999.

Skotko, Brian. "Prenatally Diagnosed Down Syndrome: Mothers Who Continued Their Pregnancies Evaluate Their Health Care Providers." *American Journal of Obstetrics and Gynecology* 192, no. 3 (March 2005).

Staub, Debbie. *Delicate Threads: Friendships Between Children With and Without Special Needs in Inclusive Settings.* Bethesda, MD: Woodbine House, 1998.

"Survey: Down Syndrome Diagnoses Found Wanting, Seven Specific Recommendations Offered." *Harvard Gazette*, March 3, 2005.

Trisomy 21 Online Community; www.trisomy21online.com/.

Uno Mas! Bulletin Board; http://unomas.proboards10.com/index.cgi/.

Winders. *Gross Motor Skills.*

Zuckoff, Mitchell. *Choosing Naia: A Family's Journey.* Boston: Beacon Press, 2002.

# Glossary of Terms

ADVOCATE a person who takes action to help another; also, to take action on one's own behalf

AGES AND STAGES QUESTIONNAIRE (ASQ) a set of questions for parents used to help determine if a child is achieving age-appropriate milestones

ALPHA-FETOPROTEIN (AFP) a protein in a pregnant woman's blood that is used as a screening tool for the possible presence of genetic conditions

AMERICAN SIGN LANGUAGE (ASL) a language system that uses two hands for making gestures to communicate

AMERICANS WITH DISABILITIES ACT (ADA) a law that prohibits discrimination by government agencies and employers against people with learning differences and physical differences

AMNIOCENTESIS (AMNIO) a method of prenatal testing in which a needle is inserted into the womb and a small amount of fluid is withdrawn

APNEA OF PREMATURITY when premature infants stop breathing for fifteen to twenty seconds during sleep

APRAXIA also sometimes called developmental verbal apraxia; a condition in which children have the ability to make the oral motor movements for speech but have difficulty putting them together in the correct sequence

ASSESSMENT a professional evaluation of a child's developmental strengths and weaknesses

ATLANTOAXIAL INSTABILITY a fault in the joints of the upper bones of the spinal column, revealed through X-rays

AT RISK children who have, or could have, problems with their development

ATRIAL SEPTAL DEFECT (ASD) a hole in the wall between the two upper chambers of the heart

ATRIOVENTRICULAR CANAL DEFECT (AV CANAL) a condition that affects the walls between the two upper chambers and the two lower chambers of the heart

AUDIOLOGIST a person trained to measure and evaluate hearing

AUDITORY BRAINSTEM RESPONSE (ABR) also known as BAER or ABER; a method for electronically measuring the brain's response to sound

AVENT a brand of breast pump used for hand-expressing breast milk

BILATERAL COORDINATION the efficient use of both sides of the body during an activity

BRADYCARDIA a repeated drop in heart rate below eighty beats per minute

BRUSHFIELD SPOTS light or white dots in the iris

CAFCIT brand name of an oral caffeine solution sometimes given to premature infants who are having trouble breathing

CAMPTODACTYLY a permanent bend in one or both of the small joints in a finger, often the pinky

CARDIOLOGIST a doctor who specializes in diagnosing and treating heart conditions

CELIAC DISEASE a genetic sensitivity to gluten, a protein found in wheat, barley, oats, and rye, that prevents the absorption of energy and nutrients from all food

CERTIFICATE OF CLINICAL COMPETENCE IN SPEECH-LANGUAGE PATHOLOGY (CCC-SLP) a professional credential for speech-language pathologists awarded by the American Speech-Language-Hearing Association

CESAREAN SECTION (C-SECTION) a surgical procedure where an incision is made in the abdomen and uterus, through which the baby is delivered

CHROMOSOMES rod-shaped cones that hold genetic material from both the mother and the father

COGNITIVE DEVELOPMENT a baby's emerging skills for perceiving, understanding, and remembering information

COLIC an uncontrollable, unexplained crying in infants

CONDITIONED PLAY AUDIOMETRY (CPA) a method of testing hearing that uses sounds and play as a reward

CONGENITAL HEART DEFECTS (CHD) heart problems present at birth

CYTOGENETICIST a doctor who studies chromosomes

DECIBEL a measurement of sound level

DEOXYRIBONUCLEIC ACID (DNA) the spiral-shaped molecules that carry genes

DEVELOPMENTAL MILESTONE a skill or set of skills in relationship to the time period in which they are acquired

DISJUNCTION the separation of chromosomes during initial cell development

DOWN SYNDROME (DS OR T21) the most commonly occurring genetic condition, in which there is extra material at the twenty-first chromosome, also known as trisomy 21

DYSARTHRIA difficulty with oral motor skills that affect speech

EAR, NOSE AND THROAT PHYSICIAN (ENT) a doctor who specializes in the ear, nose, and throat areas of the body

EAR TUBES small tubes surgically implanted in the eardrum to allow fluid to drain away; also referred to as Pressure Equalization (PE) tubes

EARLY INTERVENTION programs that vary by state for children from birth to age three who show a significant delay or disorder in development, or have a condition that is known to keep them from developing as expected

EARLY LEARNING ACCOMPLISHMENT PROFILE (E-LAP) a booklet containing a checklist of age-appropriate skills and achievements, which is sometimes used in evaluations

ECHOCARDIOGRAM (EKG) a test that creates an ultrasound image of the heart

EVALUATION a professional assessment of skills and strengths, as well as deficits and weaknesses, in relationship to a peer group

EXPRESSIVE LANGUAGE SKILLS the ability to use gestures, words and/or writing to communicate one's intent

FAMILY SUPPORT SERVICES (FSS) programs that vary by state to help families support their child with a disability in their home

FINE MOTOR SKILLS the ability to perform movements using the small muscles of the body, especially fingers and toes

FLUORESCENCE IN SITU HYBRIDIZATION (FISH) TEST a technique that uses a specific protein designed to stick to unique DNA in a cell, for examination under a microscope

Follow Along Services (FAS) programs that vary by state to monitor infants and toddlers who are at risk for developmental delays

Frequency a measurement of sound waves

Gastroesophageal reflux disease (GERD) the involuntary transfer of stomach contents into the esophagus

Genes microscopic forms that contain hereditary material from both the mother and the father

Gestation the period of development in the uterus from conception until birth, usually thirty-seven to forty-two weeks

Gross motor skills actions that require use of the large muscles of the body, like rolling, sitting, crawling, walking, and running

Hyperextension straightening of the joint beyond normal limits, sometimes called double-jointed

Hypotonia a low degree of tension in the muscles, also called low-tone

Immunization building resistance to particular diseases through a schedule of vaccinations

In vitro fertilization (IVF) implantation of fertilized eggs in a woman's uterus

Individualized education program (IEP) a written program for the education of a child aged three to twenty-one who's receiving Special Education services from school districts

Individual Family Services Plan (IFSP) a written program explaining the services and goals for families with infants who have developmental delays

Individuals with Disabilities Education Act (IDEA) a law that establishes the rights of all children to an appropriate public education

INTELLIGENCE QUOTIENT (IQ) a numerical measurement of intelligence as derived from standardized tests

ISOLETTE a brand name for an incubator that keeps the baby warm with moistened air in a clean environment and helps to protect the baby from noise and drafts

KARYOTYPE a photograph of a person's number and arrangement of chromosomes

LEUKEMIA a type of cancer that attacks red blood cells

LOVE AND LEARNING a multisensory approach to reading created by Joe and Sue Kotlinski

MEDELA a brand of breast pump that electronically expresses breast milk

MEDICAID a federal program that provides medical assistance to people with a proven financial need

MEDICARE a federal program providing payments for medical care for people with a proven financial need

MICROCEPHALY a smaller than usual head circumference

MORE WHISTLES whistles used in a program designed by Sara Rosenfield-Johnson in which a hierarchy of horns are used to develop oral motor skills

MOSAICISM a rare type of Down syndrome where the trisomy is present in some, but not all, of a person's cells

NEONATAL INTENSIVE CARE UNIT (NICU) a unit of a hospital specializing in the care of ill or premature newborn infants

NONDISJUNCTION TRISOMY 21 the most common form of Down syndrome, in which the twenty-first chromosome does not separate from itself evenly

NUTRITIONIST a person with specialized training in diet and nutrition

NUTRIVENE-D a nutrition-related vitamin therapy program based on a formula created by Dixie Lawrence Tafoya, marketed by International Nutrition, Inc.

OBJECT PERMANENCE a cognitive milestone marked by the understanding that an object continues to exist even when it's out of sight

OCCUPATIONAL THERAPY (OT) activities used to encourage the development of fine motor skills and the integration of information from all five senses (sight, sound, taste, touch, and smell)

OPHTHALMOLOGIST a doctor who specializes in diagnosing and treating conditions of the eyes

ORAL MOTOR SKILLS the ability to use the muscles in and around the mouth for chewing, swallowing, drinking, and speaking

ORTHOTICS devices used to help aid the development of the feet, ankles, and legs

OTITIS MEDIA inflammation of the middle ear, also called an ear infection

OTOACOUSTIC EMISSION TESTING (OAE) a test that measures emissions from the middle ear and is used to screen for middle-ear problems

PALMAR GRASP a way of handling objects using fingers and the palm of the hand

PARENT EATING AND NUTRITION ASSESSMENT FOR CHILDREN WITH SPECIAL HEALTH NEEDS (PEACH) a survey written for parents in order to identify children who need feeding assistance

PATENT DUCTUS ARTERIOSUS (PDA) a condition in which the ductus arteriosus remains open after birth; PDAs often close by themselves, but require monitoring

PEDIATRIC INTENSIVE CARE UNIT (PICU) a unit of the hospital where infants and children are provided intensive care for illness or injury

PEOPLE FIRST LANGUAGE a method of speaking about individuals with learning differences or physical differences that puts the person first and the medical diagnosis second

PHYSICAL THERAPY activities that encourage development of the large muscles

PICTURE EXCHANGE COMMUNICATION SYSTEM (PECS) a technique for teaching a child that communication can be used to satisfy wants and needs, originally developed by Andy Bondy and Lori Frost

PINCER GRASP a developmental milestone achieved when a child uses the thumb and index finger to pick up small objects

PULMONARY ARTERIAL HYPERTENSION (PAH) high blood pressure in the pulmonary artery, also known as pulmonary hypertension (PH)

RECEPTIVE LANGUAGE SKILLS the ability to understand the gestures, speech, and written communication of others

REGRESSION the loss of developmental skills

RESPITE CARE child care provided to allow parents time away from their children with learning or physical disabilities

SEIZURE a convulsion or loss of consciousness resulting from unusual electrical activity in the brain

SELF-HELP SKILLS the ability to take care of one's basic needs, including bathing, grooming, dressing, and eating

SENSORY INTEGRATION SKILLS the ability to receive information from the five senses (sight, sound, smell, touch, and taste) and process it in a meaningful way

SIGNED EXACT ENGLISH SYSTEM (SEE) a sign language system that uses gestures to duplicate the spoken English language

SOCIAL SECURITY DISABILITY INSURANCE (SSDI) a federal program that provides financial aid to people with a qualifying disability

SOCIAL SKILLS the ability to function in groups of people

SPEECH the process of producing voice and sound combinations in a verbal language

SPEECH-LANGUAGE PATHOLOGIST (SLP) a person with specialized training in communication, language, and speech

SPEECH THERAPY (ST) activities that encourage the development of oral motor skills and expressive and receptive language

SUDDEN INFANT DEATH SYNDROME (SIDS) the sudden and unexplained death of an infant who is younger than one year old

SUPPLEMENTAL SECURITY INCOME (SSI) Social Security benefits for children under the age of eighteen who have disabilities

TAX EQUITY AND FISCAL RESPONSIBILITY ACT (TEFRA) legislation that provides medical assistance to some disabled children who live at home with their families, based on the child's disability and not parental income

TISSUE TRANSGLUTAMINASE TEST (IgA-tTG) a blood test that is the preferred method for screening for celiac disease

THYROID a gland in the neck that produces a hormone that regulates metabolism

TRANSLOCATION TRISOMY 21 a rare form of Down syndrome caused when part of the extra number 21 chromosome breaks off and attaches itself elsewhere

TRANSVERSE PALMAR CREASE a single crease across the palm that occurs in some children with Down syndrome

**TRIPLE SCREEN** a maternal blood test at weeks sixteen to eighteen of pregnancy for the screening of markers for some genetic disorders, including Down syndrome

**TRIPOD GRASP** holding an object, such as a crayon, using the thumb, second, and third fingers

**TOTAL COMMUNICATION** the combined use of signs or gestures with sounds and words to facilitate the development of communication skills

**TYMPANOMETRY** a test for middle-ear fluid and middle-ear pressure that measures the eardrum as it transmits sound

**U-SERIES** an early vitamin therapy program created by Dr. Henry Turkel

**ULTRASOUND** the use of sound waves to create an image of the inside of the body

**UMBILICAL HERNIA** a protrusion of the navel caused by incomplete development of the stomach muscles

**VENTRICULAR SEPTAL DEFECT (VSD)** a hole between the two lower walls of the heart

**VESTIBULAR** relating to the sensory system located in the inner ear that enables the body to maintain balance

**VISUAL MOTOR SKILLS** the ability to use the eyes to guide hand movements

**VISUAL REINFORCEMENT AUDIOMETRY (VRA)** a method of testing hearing using sound cues and visual reinforcement

**VOCATIONAL TRAINING** job training for a specific vocation

# Resources

**Books and Pamphlets for Parents and Professionals**

Accardo, Pasquale J., and Barbara Y. Whitman, eds. *Dictionary of Developmental Disabilities Terminology, 2nd ed.* Baltimore: Paul H. Brookes Publishing Co., 2003.

A comprehensive guide to terms and definitions, with illustrations. Includes a CD-ROM.

Bakely, Donald. *Bethy and the Mouse: A Father Remembers His Children with Disabilities.* Cambridge, MA: Brookline Books, 1997.

A father's recollections of life with two of his children.

————. *Down Syndrome: One Family's Journey.* Cambridge, MA: Brookline Books, 2002.

A father's story of the life of his daughter Beth, who was born with Down syndrome.

Baskin, Amy, and Heather Fawcett. *More Than a Mom: Living a Full and Balanced Life When Your Child Has Special Needs.* Bethesda, MD: Woodbine House, 2006.

A practical guide written by two moms of children with learning differences.

Batshaw, Mark L., ed. *When Your Child Has a Disability: The Complete Sourcebook of Daily and Medical Care*, rev. ed. Baltimore: Paul H. Brookes Publishing Co., 2001.

A collection of essays that gives a general overview of many different diagnoses.

Beck, Martha. *Expecting Adam: A True Story of Birth, Rebirth and Everyday Magic.* New York: Crown Publishing Group, 1998.

One woman's story of coming to terms with her prenatal diagnosis of Down syndrome.

Bérubé, Michael. *Life As We Know It: A Father, a Family, and an Exceptional Child.* New York: Knopf, 1996.

A father looks at what life with his son has taught him, especially about intelligence.

Bruni, Maryanne. *Fine Motor Skills for Children with Down Syndrome: A Guide for Parents and Professionals*, 2nd ed. Bethesda, MD: Woodbine House, 2006.

A practical guide to encouraging the development of fine motor skills written by a licensed occupational therapist and mother to a daughter with Down syndrome.

Buck, Pearl S. *The Child Who Never Grew*, 2nd ed. Bethesda, MD: Woodbine House, 1992.

Pulitzer and Nobel prize–winning author's story of her daughter, born with phenylketonuria, which went undiagnosed during her lifetime.

Burke, Chris, and J. B. McDaniel. *A Special Kind of Hero: Chris Burke's Own Story.* Lincoln, NE: iUniverse, 2001.

Actor and self-advocate Chris Burke writes about his life.

Carroll, Bruce. *Sometimes Miracles Hide*. New York: Simon and Schuster, 2003.

A collection of letters written in response to the hit song by the same title.

Carter, Erik W. *Including People with Disabilities in Faith Communities: A Guide for Service Providers, Families, and Congregations*. Baltimore: Paul H. Brookes Publishing Co., 2007.

A guidebook of strategies, including forms to photocopy, for inclusion in faith-based communities.

Cohen, William I., Lynn Nadel, and Myra E. Madnick, eds. *Down Syndrome: Visions for the 21st Century*. New York: Wiley-Liss, Inc., 2002.

A collection of essays by experts, including parents.

Coleman, Jeanine G. *The Early Intervention Dictionary: A Multidisciplinary Guide to Terminology*, 3rd ed. Bethesda, MD: Woodbine House, 2006.

An extensive guide to abbreviations, definitions, and terminology.

Cunningham, Cliff. *Understanding Down Syndrome: An Introduction for Parents*. Cambridge, MA: Brookline Books, 1996.

An overview of Down syndrome by a British lecturer and physician.

Dunst, Carl J., Carol M. Trivette, and Angela G. Deal. *Supporting and Strengthening Families: Methods, Strategies and Practices* (vol. 1, 1994; vol. 2, 1995). Cambridge, MA: Brookline Books, 1994.

A collection of papers researching strategies for building strong families.

Dybwad, Gunnar, and Hank Bersani, Jr. *New Voices: Self-Advocacy by People with Disabilities.* Cambridge, MA: Brookline Books, 1998.

A collection of essays examining the status of self-advocacy activities by people with developmental disabilites.

Edwards, Kim. *The Memory Keeper's Daughter.* New York: Viking, 2005.

A fictional account of a father who secretly gives away his twin daughter with Down syndrome in the 1960s.

Falvey, M. *Believe in My Child with Special Needs!: Helping Children Achieve Their Potential in School.* Baltimore: Brookes Publishing, 2005.

A practical guide to strategies for success in the school setting, written by an educator and mom of a child with learning differences.

Gill, Barbara. *Changed by a Child: Companion Notes for Parents of a Child with a Disability.* Garden City, NY: Doubleday, 1997.

A collection of short inspiring anecdotes by a mother of a child with Down syndrome.

Glover, M. E, J. L. Preminger, and A. R. Sanford. *Early LAP: The Early Learning Accomplishment Profile for Young Children, Birth to 36 Months.* Chapel Hill, NC: Chapel Hill Training-Outreach Project, 1988.

A booklet for scoring early learning achievements.

Goode, David, ed. *Quality of Life for Persons with Disabilities: International Perspectives and Issues.* Cambridge, MA: Brookline Books, 1994.

A global look at quality-of-life issues as people with learning and physical differences live, work, play, and go to school.

Greenstein, Doreen, et al. *Backyards and Butterflies: Ways to Include Children with Disabilities in Outdoor Activities.* Cambridge, MA: Brookline Books, 1995.

Tips and suggestions for including your child in everyday activities.

Hassold, T. J., and D. Patterson, eds. *Down Syndrome: A Promising Future, Together.* New York: John Wiley & Sons, 1999.

A comprehensive overview by experts, including parents.

Horstmeier, DeAnna. *Teaching Math to People with Down Syndrome and other Hands-On Learners.* Bethesda, MD: Woodbine House, 2004.

A practical guide for teaching everyday math skills.

Jobling, Anne, and Naznin Virji-Babul. *Down Syndrome: Play, Move, and Grow.* Vancouver, BC: Down Syndrome Research Foundation, 2004.

Tips and suggestions for ways to encourage and support movement.

Josephson, Gretchen, and Allen C. Crocker, ed. *Bus Girl: Poems by Gretchen Josephson.* Cambridge, MA: Brookline Books, 1997.

Poems written over the course of several decades by a woman with Down syndrome.

Kidder, Cynthia, Brian Skotko, and K. Dew, eds. *Common Threads: Celebrating Life with Down Syndrome.* Rochester Hills, MI: Band of Angels Press, 2001.

A book of photographs and personal essays by families of children with Down syndrome.

Kingsley, Jason, and Mitchell Levitz. *Count Us In: Growing Up with Down Syndrome*, rev. ed. New York: Harcourt Brace & Company, 2007.

Two friends—coauthors and self-advocates—write about living with Down syndrome.

Klein, Stanley, Ph.D., and John Kemp, eds. *Reflections from a Different Journey: What Adults with Disabilities Wish All Parents Knew.* New York: McGraw-Hill Companies, 2004.

Forty essays written by adults with disabilities discussing the positive and negative aspects of their growing-up years.

Klein, Stanley, Ph.D., and Kim Schive, eds. *You Will Dream New Dreams: Inspiring Personal Stories by Parents of Children with Disabilities.* New York: Kensington Books, 2001.

A collection of personal writing by parents of children with learning and physical differences.

Kumin, Libby. *Early Communication Skills for Children with Down Syndrome: A Guide for Parents and Professionals.* Bethesda, MD: Woodbine House, 2003.

A practical guide for encouraging the development of communication skills.

La Leche League International. *The Womanly Art of Breastfeeding*, 6th rev. ed. Schaumburg, IL: La Leche League International, 1997.

A practical guide to breast-feeding.

Lavin, Judith Loseff. *Special Kids Need Special Parents: A Resource for Parents of Children with Special Needs.* New York: Penguin Group, 2001.

A practical guide drawn from interviews with health-care professionals and parents, by the mother of a child with developmental differences.

Lott, Brett. *Jewel.* New York: Pocket Books, 1999.

A fictional story of a mother raising her daughter born with Down syndrome in 1943.

MacLeod, Kent. *Down Syndrome and Vitamin Therapy.* Baltimore: Kemanso Publishing Ltd., 2003.

A discussion of vitamin therapy by an author affiliated with Nutri-Chem.

McGuire, Dennis, and Brian Chicoine. *Mental Wellness in Adults with Down Syndrome: A Guide to Emotional and Behavioral Strengths and Challenges.* Bethesda, MD: Woodbine House, 2006.

A practical guide to supporting emotional wellness in adults with Down syndrome.

MacDonell Mandema, J. *Family Makers: Joyful Lives with Down Syndrome.* Menlo Park, CA: The Mandema Family Foundation, 2002.

A book of black-and-white photos and personal essays celebrating family life with Down syndrome.

Marino, B., and Siegfried M. Pueschel, eds. *Heart Disease in Persons with Down Syndrome.* Baltimore: Paul H. Brookes Publishing Co., 1996.

An in-depth explanation of heart disease as it occurs in people with Down syndrome.

Marshak, Laura E., and Fran P. Prezant. *Married with Special-Needs Children: A Couple's Guide to Keeping Connected.* Bethesda, MD: Woodbine House, 2007.

A practical guide in which the authors draw on their combined professional experience in marital counseling and parent training, in addition to the experience and advice of other parents.

Medlen, Joan Guthrie. *The Down Syndrome Nutrition Handbook*. Lake Oswego, OR: Phronesis Publishing, 2006.

A practical guide to diet and nutrition by a licensed dietician and mother of a son with Down syndrome.

Meyer, D. J., ed. *Uncommon Fathers: Reflections on Raising a Child with a Disability*. Rockville, MD: Woodbine House, 1995.

A collection of personal writings by fathers of children with developmental differences.

Miller, Jon F., Mark Leddy, and Lewis A. Leavitt, eds. *Improving the Communication of People with Down Syndrome*. Baltimore: Paul H. Brookes Publishing Co., 1999.

A practical guide to speech development, edited by three physicians.

Miller, Nancy B. *Everybody's Different: Understanding and Changing Our Reactions to Disabilities*. Baltimore: Paul H. Brookes Publishing Co., 1999.

A practical guide for people to become more comfortable with and accepting of disability.

———. *Nobody's Perfect: Living and Growing with Children Who Have Special Needs*. Baltimore: Paul H. Brookes Publishing Co., 1994.

A practical guide to the emotions of being a parent of a child with a learning or physical difference.

MPRRC. "A Primer on People First Language." Logan, UT: Mountain Plains Regional Resource Center, 1999.

A description of language that puts the individual ahead of the diagnosis.

Naseef, Robert A. *Special Children, Challenged Parents: The Struggles and Rewards of Raising a Child with a Disability.* Baltimore: Paul H. Brookes Publishing Co., 2001.

A practical guide to the challenges of raising a child with developmental differences, written by a father of a son with autism.

NDSS. "Down Syndrome: Myths and Truths." New York: National Down Syndrome Society, 1999.

Common misconceptions about Down syndrome corrected.

———. "A Promising Future Together: A Guide for New and Expectant Parents." New York: National Down Syndrome Society, 2003.

A 39-page overview of the supports and services recommended by the NDSS.

Noble, Vicki. *Down Is Up for Aaron Eagle: A Mother's Spiritual Journey with Down Syndrome.* New York: HarperCollins, 1993.

A mother's story of spiritual growth because of her son with Down sydnrome.

Oelwein, P. *Teaching Reading to Children with Down Syndrome: A Guide for Parents and Teachers.* Bethesda, MD: Woodbine House, 1995.

A practical guide to teaching reading to children with Down syndrome, and other visual learners.

Palmer, Greg. *Adventures in the Mainstream: Coming of Age with Down Syndrome.* Bethesda, MD: Woodbine House, 2005.

A father's description of life with his adult son with Down syndrome.

Pueschel, Siegfried M. *A Parent's Guide to Down Syndrome: Toward a Brighter Future.* Baltimore: Paul H. Brookes Publishing Co., 1990.

A collection of writing by professionals giving an overview of raising a child with Down syndrome.

Rogers, Dale Evans. *Angel Unaware,* rep. ed. Tarrytown, NY: Fleming H. Revell, 1992.

A father's story of his love for his child with Down syndrome.

Rothman, Barbara Katz. *The Book of Life: A Personal and Ethical Guide to Race, Normality, and the Implications of the Human Genome Project.* Boston: Beacon Press, 2000.

A look at genetic research, testing, and the social cost of both.

Santelli, Betsy, Florence Stewart Poyadue, and Jane Leora Young, eds. *The Parent to Parent Handbook: Connecting Families of Children with Special Needs.* Baltimore: Paul H. Brookes Publishing Co., 2001.

A practical guide for parents and professionals interested in building parent-to-parent support groups.

Schwartz, Susan, and Joan E. Heller Miller. *The New Language of Toys: Teaching Communication Skills to Children with Special Needs, A Guide for Parents and Teachers.* Bethesda, MD: Woodbine House, 1996.

A practical guide to toys that facilitate learning through play.

Schwier, Karin Melberg, and Erin Schwier Stewart. *Breaking Bread, Nourishing Connections: People with and without Disabilities Together at Mealtime*. Baltimore: Paul H. Brookes Publishing Co., 2005.

A guide to mealtimes, including practical strategies, as well as personal essays, poems, and photographs.

Siegel, Bryna, and Stuart C. Silverstein. *What About Me? Growing Up with a Developmentally Disabled Sibling*. Cambridge, MA: Da Capo, 2001.

A guide for parents describing possible sibling reactions, and suggestions for encouraging healthy sibling relationships.

Soper, Kathryn Lynard. *Gifts: Mothers Reflect on How Children With Down Syndrome Enrich Their Lives*. Bethesda, MD: Woodbine House, 2007.

Sixty-three personal essays written by mothers of children with Down syndrome, with a foreword by parenting expert Martha Sears, also a mother of a son with Down syndrome.

Staub, Debbie. *Delicate Threads: Friendships Between Children With and Without Special Needs in Inclusive Settings*. Bethesda, MD: Woodbine House, 1998.

A practical guide to building and sustaining children's friendships.

Stray-Gundersen, Karen, ed. *Babies with Down Syndrome: A New Parents' Guide*, 2nd ed. Bethesda, MD: Woodbine House, 1995.

A collection of practical essays by experts in Down syndrome for new parents.

Sumar, Sonia. *Yoga for the Special Child: A Therapeutic Approach for Infants and Children with Down Syndrome, Cerebral*

*Palsy, and Learning Disabilities.* Buckingham, VA: Special Yoga Publications, 1998.

A practical guide to encouraging body movement and beginning yoga practice.

Trainer, Marilyn. *Differences in Common: Straight Talk on Mental Retardation, Down Syndrome, and Life.* Bethesda, MD: Woodbine House, 1991.

A mother's thoughts on raising her child with Down syndrome.

Van Dyke, D. C., Philip Mattheis, Susan Schoon Eberly, and Janet Williams, eds. *Medical and Surgical Care for Children with Down Syndrome: A Guide for Parents.* Bethesda, MD: Woodbine House, 1995.

A practical guide for parents of children with medical issues.

Voss, Kimberly S. *Teaching by Design: Using Your Computer to Create Materials for Students with Learning Differences.* Bethesda, MD: Woodbine House, 2005.

A practical guide for parents and teachers to developing curriculum; includes a CD-ROM.

Vredevelt, Pam. *Angel Behind the Rocking Chair.* New York: Waterbrook Press, 1998.

A book of personal, faith-based essays by a mother of a child with Down syndrome.

Wenig, Marsha. *YogaKids: Educating the Whole Child Through Yoga.* Michigan City, IN: YogaKids, 1991.

A practical guide to more than fifty yoga poses, paired with activities to stimulate verbal, spatial, and artistic skills.

Winders, Patricia C. *Gross Motor Skills in Children with Down Syndrome: A Guide for Parents and Professionals.* Bethesda, MD: Woodbine House, 1997.

A practical guide to encouraging gross motor development.

Zuckoff, Mitchell. *Choosing Naia: A Family's Journey.* Boston: Beacon Press, 2002.

One family's story, as told by a journalist, of their prenatal diagnosis of Down syndrome.

## Books for Young Children

Bednarczyk, Angela, and Janet Weinstock. *Opposites: A Beginner's Book of Signs.* Long Island City, NY: Star Bright Books, 1996.

A beginning book of American Sign Language, also available in Spanish.

———. *Happy Birthday.* Long Island City, NY: Star Bright Books, 1996.

A beginning book of American Sign Language.

Bouwkamp, Julie. *Hi, I'm Ben! . . . and I've Got a Secret!,* 2nd ed. Rochester Hills, MI: Band of Angels Press, 2007.

Everyday life with a little boy with Down syndrome, told with words and photographs.

Brown, Tricia. *Someone Special, Just Like You* (an Owlet Book). New York: Henry Holt & Co., 1995.

Photographs of children doing everyday activities in an inclusive preschool.

Bunnett, Rochelle. *Friends at School.* Long Island City, NY: Star Bright Books, 2005.

Children of mixed abilities at school, told with words and photographs, also available in Spanish.

Cairo, Shelley. *Our Brother Has Down's Syndrome: An Introduction for Children.* Toronto, Canada: Annick Press Ltd., 2002.

Two older sisters share what it's like having a little brother with Down syndrome through words and photographs.

Carter, Alden R. *Big Brother Dustin.* Morton Grove, IL: Albert Whitman & Company, 1997.

The story of Dustin, a boy with Down syndrome, who learns how to be a big brother, as told with words and photographs, for grades preschool to third.

Christian, Cheryl. *Where Does It Go?* Long Island City, NY: Star Bright Books, 2005.

A lift-the-flap board book featuring children of mixed abilities, available in multiple languages, including Spanish, for children ages birth–4.

———. *Where's the Puppy?* Long Island City, NY: Star Bright Books, 2005.

A lift-the-flap board book featuring a puppy, available in multiple languages, including Spanish, for children ages birth–4.

DeBear, Kirsten. *Be Quiet, Marina!* Long Island City, NY: Star Bright Books, 2001.

The friendship between two three-year-old girls, one with Down syndrome and one with cerebral palsy, told in words and photographs, for ages 3–8.

Dwight, Laura. *Brothers and Sisters.* Long Island City, NY: Star Bright Books, 2005.

The story of several family groups living and playing together, as told with words and photographs, for ages 4–8.

———. *We Can Do It!* Long Island City, NY: Star Bright Books, 1998.

Photographs of five children with learning and physical differences having fun and enjoying ordinary activities at home and at school, for ages 4–8.

Ely, Lesley. *Looking After Louis.* Morton Grove, IL: Albert Whitman & Company, 2004.

The story of a boy with autism in an inclusive classroom, for children in grades 1–4.

Fenton, Anne Lobock. *Tikun Olam.* Cambridge, MA: Brookline Books, 1997.

A children's picture book about a Mr. Fixit who tries to fix his sick friend.

Girnis, Margaret. *1 2 3 for You and Me.* Morton Grove, IL: Albert Whitman and Co., 2001.

A counting book featuring photographs of children with Down syndrome.

———. *ABC for You and Me.* Morton Grove, IL: Albert Whitman and Co., 2000.

Photographs of kids with Down syndrome making letters with their bodies.

L.A. Goal. *Disabled Fables.* Long Island City, NY: Star Bright Books, 2005.

Aesop's fables as interpreted through the eyes of artists with developmental differences, with a foreword by Sean Penn.

Maguire, Arlene. *Special People, Special Ways.* Arlington, TX: Future Horizons, 2001.

Commonalities are emphasized in this illustrated rhyming book for children ages 4–8.

Pitzer, Marjorie W. *I Can, Can You?* Bethesda, MD: Woodbine House, 2005.

A board book of photographs of children with Down syndrome doing everyday activities, ages birth–4.

Rabe, Bernice. *Where's Chimpy?* Morton Grove, IL: Albert Whitman & Company, 1991.

A child with Down syndrome and her father retrace the day with the hopes of finding a beloved stuffed animal, for preschoolers to grade two.

Rogers, Fred. *Let's Talk About It: Extraordinary Friends.* New York: Putnam, 2000.

The author, the children's television personality Mister Rogers, discusses learning and physical differences and how they make us feel, for children in grades 1–3.

Rickert, Janet Elizabeth. *Russ and the Firehouse.* Bethesda, MD: Woodbine House, 1999.

The story of Russ, a five-year-old with Down syndrome, and his day at the firehouse, told with words and photographs, for ages 3–7.

Stuve-Bodeen, Stephanie. *The Best Worst Brother.* Bethesda, MD: Woodbine House, 2005.

A big sister's view of her relationship with her younger brother, who has Down syndrome, for ages 3–8. Illustrated by Charlotte Fremaux.

———. *We'll Paint the Octopus Red.* Bethesda, MD: Woodbine House, 1998.

A father reassures his daughter after the birth of a baby with Down syndrome, for ages 3–7. Illustrated by Pam DeVito.

Tomas, Pat. *Don't Call Me Special: A First Look at Disability.* Hauppauge, NY: Barron's Educational Series, 2005.

The author, a therapist and counselor, encourages children to think and ask questions, for children ages 3–8. With illustrations by Lesley Harker.

Thrasher, Amy. *My Friend Isabelle Teacher's Guide.* Bethesda, MD: Woodbine House, 2004.

A guide to using Eliza Woloson's book *My Friend Isabelle* as a teaching tool in inclusive settings.

Willis, Jeanne. *Susan Laughs.* New York: Henry Holt & Co., 2000.

The story of a child who uses a wheelchair, as told through simple rhymes and illustrations, for grades preschool to first. Illustrations by Tony Ross.

Wojahn, Rebecca Hogue. *Evan Early.* Bethesda, MD: Woodbine House, 2006.

Siblings are reassured after the premature birth of their brother, for ages 3–7. Illustrated by Ned Gannon.

Woloson, Eliza. *My Friend Isabelle.* Bethesda, MD: Woodbine House, 2003.

A story of friendship between Charlie and Isabelle, who has Down syndrome, for ages 2–6. Illustrated by Bryan Gough.

## Books for Older Children

Hale, Natalie. *Oh Brother! Growing Up with a Special Needs Sibling*. Washington, D.C.: Magination Press, 2004.

A younger sister's story of life with her brother with Down syndrome.

Meyer, Donald J., and Patricia Vadasy. *Living with a Brother or Sister with Special Needs: A Book for Sibs*. Seattle, WA: University of Washington Press, 1996.

A practical guide for siblings.

Meyer, Donald J., ed. *The Sibling Slam Book: What It's Really Like to Have a Brother or Sister with Special Needs*. Bethesda, MD: Woodbine House, 2005.

Eighty teenagers write about their siblings.

Meyer, Donald J., and Patricia F. Vadasy. *Sibshops: Workshops for Siblings of Children with Special Needs*. Baltimore: Paul H. Brookes Publishing Co., 1994.

A guide to setting up and running a sibling workshop.

Meyer, Donald J., ed. *Views from Our Shoes: Growing Up With a Brother or Sister with Special Needs*. Bethesda, MD: Woodbine House, 1997.

Forty-five essays from children of all ages who are siblings to children with physical and learning differences.

Rue, Nancy. *Sophie's Encore* (Faithgirlz!). Grand Rapids, MI: Zonderkidz, 2006.

A young girl's baby sister, born with Down syndrome, causes her to question her faith in God.

Shriver, Maria. *What's Wrong with Timmy?* New York: Little, Brown, 2001.

A walk in the park gives a mother the opportunity to speak with her child about other children with learning and physical differences, illustrated by Sandra Speidel, for children in grades 3–5.

## DVDs and Videos

ABC Television, *Nightline* with Ted Koppel. "Mother's Mission." VHS. December 1996.

A look at targeted nutritional intervention, featuring Dixie Lawrence Tafoya and her daughter Madison. Transcript also available.

CBS Television, *48 Hours.* "Smart Drugs for Down Syndrome: Hope or Hype?" VHS. August 21, 1997.

Erin Moriarty investigates the debate, including an interview with Dixie Lawrence Tafoya and others. Transcript available.

Allstate Insurance Company, producer. *Gifts of Love.* VHS. New York: National Down Syndrome Society, 2000.

Four families of children with Down syndrome talk about their feelings and experiences.

Coleman, Rachel. *Signing Time! Volume 1: My First Signs.* VHS & DVD. Salt Lake City: Two Little Hands Productions, 2002.

Adults and children teach sign language skills through songs, words, and play.

————. *Signing Time! Volume 2: Playtime Signs.* VHS & DVD. Salt Lake City: Two Little Hands Productions, 2002.

Adults and children teach sign language skills through songs, words, and play.

————. *Signing Time! Volume3: Everyday Signs.* VHS & DVD. Salt Lake City: Two Little Hands Productions, 2002.

Adults and children teach sign language skills through songs, words, and play.

Connecticut Down Syndrome Congress. *Life with Down Syndrome.* VHS. Hartford, CT: Connecticut Down Syndrome Congress, 1997.

Everyday life with families of children with Down syndrome at various ages.

Down Syndrome Association of Central Ohio. *Like Any Child, Raising a Child with Down Syndrome.* VHS. Worthington, OH: Down Syndrome Association of Central Ohio, 1997.

Parents, professionals, and people with Down syndrome talk about everyday life, including an interview with Chris Burke.

Endless Horizon Productions. *Emma's Gifts.* DVD. Charlotte, NC: Endless Horizon Productions, 2003.

Everyday life with fraternal twins Emma and Abigail, as told by their parents, through the preschool years and including IEP planning.

Gibbs, Betsy, and Ann Springer. *Early Use of Total Communication. Parents' Perspectives on Using Sign Language with Young Children with Down Syndrome.* VHS. Baltimore: Paul H. Brookes, 1993.

A practical guide to the total communication approach of simultaneously using speech and sign language.

Goodwin, Thomas C., and Geraldine Wurzburg, for Home Box Office. *Educating Peter*. VHS. New York: Insight Media, Inc., 1992.

Academy Award–winning short-subject film about a year in the life of a child with Down syndrome in an inclusive school setting. Includes a seven-page study guide.

Graves, Duane, director. *Up Syndrome*. VHS. Austin, TX: Trisomy Films, 2000.

Award-winning documentary of a year in the life of the director's childhood friend, who was born with Down syndrome.

Hanlon, Grace M., producer. *Successfully Parenting Your Baby with Special Needs: Early Intervention for Ages Birth to Three*. VHS. Baltimore: Paul H. Brooks, 1999.

A practical guide for new parents featuring advice from other parents and professionals.

Karen Gaffney Foundation. *Journey of a Lifetime . . . Beginning with the End in Mind*. VHS. Portland, OR: The Karen Gaffney Foundation, 1998.

A practical guide for new parents with information about early intervention.

Kemper National Insurance Co., underwriters. *Opportunities to Grow*. VHS. New York: National Down Syndrome Society, 1992.

Sequel to *Gifts of Love*, featuring people with Down syndrome ages six to twenty-six, including Andrea Friedman, Chris Burke, John Taylor, and Jason Kingsley.

Kotlinski, Joe and Sue. *Love and Learning.* VHS, DVD, CD, and audiocassette. Dearborn, MI: Love and Learning, 1989.

A multisensory approach to teaching reading.

Kumin, Libby. *What Did You Say? A Guide to Speech Intelligibility in People with Down Syndrome.* DVD. Directed and edited by Will Schermerhorn. Vienna, VA: Blueberry Shoes Productions, 2006.

An in-depth look at speech development by professionals.

Lamb, Karin, and Gina Lamb. *Doing Things.* VHS. Eureka, MT: Bo Peep Productions, Inc., 1988.

Typically developing children model self-help skills, such as washing, eating, and getting dressed.

———. *Sounds Around.* VHS. Eureka, MT: Bo Peep Productions, Inc., 1988.

Children with and without learning differences experience play through sounds and music.

———. *Which Way Weather?* VHS. Eureka, MT: Bo Peep Productions, Inc., 1990.

Children with and without developmental differences model appropriate weather-based activities.

Myshrall, Kate, ed. *Friends Like Me.* VHS. Worcester, MA: Massachusetts Down Syndrome Congress, 1999.

A look at the life of several people with Down syndrome, with input from siblings, friends, and classmates.

NDSS. *A Promising Future Together: A Guide for New Parents of Children with Down Syndrome.* VHS. New York: National Down Syndrome Society, 1998.

A companion to the NDSS New Parent Guide with the same title.

Owensby, Jennifer, producer and director. *The Teachings of Jon*. DVD. Durham, NC: Waking Heart Films, 2006.

A family's story of life with an adult brother with Down syndrome, as filmed by his sister.

Schermerhorn, Will. *Discovery: Pathways to Better Speech for Children with Down Syndrome*. DVD. Vienna, VA: Blueberry Shoes Productions, 2005.

A general overview of the key components to the development of speech.

———. *Down Syndrome: The First 18 Months*. DVD. Vienna, VA: Blueberry Shoes Productions, 1993.

Interviews with noted professionals and personal family stories provide an overview for new parents of children with Down syndrome.

State of the Art Productions, for Home Box Office. *Graduating Peter*. VHS & DVD. Princeton, NJ: Film for the Humanities and Sciences, 2001.

Sequel to the Academy Award–winning short-subject film *Educating Peter*.

Wenig, Marsha. *YogaKids: An Easy, Fun-filled Adventure*. DVD. Living Arts, Inc., 2000.

Children of all ages learn play through yoga to help build strength and good health.

Young, Donald, producer. *Raymond's Portrait: The Life and Art of Raymond Hu.* VHS. San Francisco: National Asian American Telecommunications Distribution, 1997.

Award-winning documentary tracing the personal and artistic development of the painter Raymond Hu, who has Down syndrome.

## National Organizations

*Disability Solutions* (newsletter)
Creating Solutions, 14535 Westlake Drive, Suite A-2, Lake Oswego, OR 97035
www.disabilitysolutions.org/

A publication for families and others interested in Down syndrome and developmental disabilities.

*Down Syndrome Quarterly* (newsletter)
www.dsrf.org/index.cfm?fuseaction-publications.dsq

An interdisciplinary journal devoted to advancing the state of knowledge about Down syndrome.

*Exceptional Parent* magazine
PO Box 3000, Denville, NJ 07834
1-800-247-8080
www.eparent.com/

Award-winning source of information, support, and outreach for parents and families of children with disabilities, and the professionals who work with them.

National Association for Down Syndrome (NADS)
www.nads.org/

An organization providing services to families and individuals with Down syndrome in the greater Chicago area. Conferences, products, and publications are available nationwide.

National Down Syndrome Congress (NDSC)
www.ndsccenter.org/

A network of local and regional groups across the country formed of parents, families, and self-advocates that holds a national convention each summer.

National Down Syndrome Society (NDSS)
666 Broadway, 8th Floor, New York, NY 10012
1-800-221-4602
www.ndss.org/

An organization created to benefit people with Down syndrome and their families through national leadership in education, research, and advocacy.

The Arc of the United States (ARC)
www.thearc.org/

The largest grassroots organization of and for people with intellectual and developmental disabilities.

## Web sites

Baby Center Bulletin Boards, Down syndrome
http://boards.babycenter.com/n/pfx/forum.aspx?webtag=bcus11985

A support board for parents of babies and children with Down syndrome.

Disability is Natural
www.disabilityisnatural.com/

A Web site for parents of babies and children with learning and physical differences.

DownSyn Forum
www.downsyn.com/

A support board for parents of babies and children with Down syndrome.

Down Syndrome: Health Issues
www.ds-health.com/

An information site maintained by Dr. Len Leshin, M.D., F.A.A.P., and father to a son with Down syndrome.

NuTriVene-D Targeted Nutritional Intervention, a Brand of International Nutrition, Inc.
www.nutrivene.com/

Product ordering information.

Pinwheels
www.jennifergrafgroneberg.com/

A blog written by Jennifer Graf Groneberg for parents of children with Down syndrome, and for the curious of heart.

Riverbend Down Syndrome Parent Support Group
www.he.net/~altonweb/cs/downsyndrome/index.htm

A Web site featuring information, links, abstracts, and a newsletter.

Trisomy 21 Online Community
www.trisomy21online.com/

A support board for parents of babies and children with Down syndrome.

Uno Mas! Bulletin Board
www.unomas21.com/

A support board for parents of babies and children with Down syndrome.

Wrightslaw

www.wrightslaw.com/

Information about special education law, education law, and advocacy for children with disabilities.

## Resources for Caregivers

Healthcare Protocol, as recommended by the NDSS
www.ndss.org/index.php?option=com_content&task=view&id=1988&Itemid=119/

Growth Charts and Head Circumference Charts, as recommended by the NDSS
www.ndss.org/index.php?option=com_content&task=view&id=603&Itemid=119/

꙳

# Welcome to Holland

*by Emily Perl Kingsley*

I am often asked to describe the experience of raising a child with a disability—to try to help people who have not shared that unique experience to understand it, to imagine how it would feel. It's like this. . . .

When you're going to have a baby, it's like planning a fabulous vacation trip—to Italy. You buy a bunch of guide books and make your wonderful plans. The Coliseum. The Michelangelo David. The gondolas in Venice. You may learn some handy phrases in Italian. It's all very exciting.

After months of eager anticipation, the day finally arrives. You pack your bags and off you go. Several hours later, the plane lands. The stewardess comes in and says, "Welcome to Holland."

*"Holland?!?"* you say. "What do you mean Holland?? I signed up for Italy! I'm supposed to be in Italy. All my life I've dreamed of going to Italy."

But there's been a change in the flight plan. They've landed in Holland and there you must stay.

The important thing is that they haven't taken you to a horrible, disgusting, filthy place, full of pestilence, famine and disease. It's just a different place.

So you must go out and buy new guide books. And you must learn a whole new language. And you will meet a whole new group of people you would never have met.

It's just a *different* place. It's slower-paced than Italy, less flashy than Italy. But after you've been there for a while and you catch your breath, you look around . . . and you begin to notice that Holland has windmills . . . and Holland has tulips. Holland even has Rembrandts.

But everyone you know is busy coming and going from Italy . . . and they're all bragging about what a wonderful time they had there. And for the rest of your life, you will say "Yes, that's where I was supposed to go. That's what I had planned."

And the pain of that will never, ever, ever, *ever* go away . . . because the loss of that dream is a very very significant loss.

But . . . if you spend your life mourning the fact that you didn't get to Italy, you may never be free to enjoy the very special, the very lovely things . . . about Holland.